Annette M. Mahoney, DSW
Editor

The Health
and Well-Being
of Caribbean Immigrants
in the United States

The Health and Well-Being of Caribbean Immigrants in the United States has been co-published simultaneously as *Journal of Immigrant & Refugee Services*, Volume 2, Numbers 3/4 2004.

Pre-publication
REVIEWS,
COMMENTARIES,
EVALUATIONS . . .

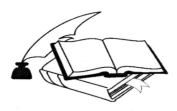

" **A** N EXCELLENT COLLECTION THAT ALL STUDENTS of the Caribbean Diaspora in particular and of development in general SHOULD READ. Despite the migration of large numbers of Caribbean nationals to North America over the past one hundred years, not much scholarly work has been done related to them and their descendents. Coming on the fortieth anniversary of the Immigration Reform Act of 1965, this book helps to fill that void. It covers a range of issues affecting Caribbean immigrants and their families in the United States."

Winston H. Griffith, PhD
Professor of Economics/Director
of the Bucknell-in-Barbados Semester
Program
Bucknell University

More Pre-publication
REVIEWS, COMMENTARIES, EVALUATIONS . . .

"A USEFUL REFERENCE RE-SOURCE FOR STUDENTS, PROVIDERS, PROFESSIONALS, AND POLICYMAKERS. . . . Interdisciplinary, comprehensive, and easy to understand. . . . This book covers critical health, social, economic, immigration, and cultural issues impacting immigrant families. It highlights the disparities in socioeconomic and health status, as well as the barriers encountered by immigrants of color in accessing health and social services. It also provides proven and insightful modalities for effectively working with this population, and presents a solid framework for shaping policy around improving service delivery for immigrants."

Elaine Reid, LCSW
Vice President
Caribbean-American Social Workers Association

"THIS HIGHLY INFORMATIVE BOOK presents a timely overview of the psychosocial issues central to the health and well-being of Caribbean immigrants in the United States. It covers critical research areas, including the impact of HIV on Caribbean communities, risk factors for infant mortality, and the protection of vulnerable populations. The breadth of topics covered makes this A VALUABLE RESOURCE FOR CLINICAL PRACTITIONERS, RESEARCHERS, AND EDUCATORS. This book is especially valuable for researchers in gender and minority health. Almost every chapter provides important insight into the unique health challenges confronted by Afro- Caribbean women. I HIGHLY RECOMMEND THIS BOOK."

John Taylor, PhD
Assistant Professor of Sociology
The Center for Demography and Population Health
Florida State University
Tallahassee

The Haworth Social Work Practice Press
An Imprint of The Haworth Press, Inc.

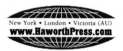

New York • London • Victoria (AU)
www.HaworthPress.com

The Health
and Well-Being
of Caribbean Immigrants
in the United States

The Health and Well-Being of Caribbean Immigrants in the United States has been co-published simultaneously as *Journal of Immigrant & Refugee Services*, Volume 2, Numbers 3/4 2004.

The *Journal of Immigrant & Refugee Services*^{TM} Monographic "Separates"

Below is a list of "separates," which in serials librarianship means a special issue simultaneously published as a special journal issue or double-issue *and* as a "separate" hardbound monograph. (This is a format which we also call a "DocuSerial.")

"Separates" are published because specialized libraries or professionals may wish to purchase a specific thematic issue by itself in a format which can be separately cataloged and shelved, as opposed to purchasing the journal on an on-going basis. Faculty members may also more easily consider a "separate" for classroom adoption.

"Separates" are carefully classified separately with the major book jobbers so that the journal tie-in can be noted on new book order slips to avoid duplicate purchasing.

You may wish to visit Haworth's website at . . .

http://www.HaworthPress.com

. . . to search our online catalog for complete tables of contents of these separates and related publications.

You may also call 1-800-HAWORTH (outside US/Canada: 607-722-5857), or Fax 1-800-895-0582 (outside US/Canada: 607-771-0012), or e-mail at:

docdelivery@haworthpress.com

The Health and Well-Being of Caribbean Immigrants in the United States, edited by Annette M. Mahoney, DSW (Vol. 2, No. 3/4, 2004). *The Health and Well-Being of Caribbean Immigrants in the United States is a timely addition to the knowledge base concerning the integration of this population into the fabric of American society. On the eve of the fortieth anniversary of the 1965 Immigration Reform Act, this book examines the relationship between immigrants from the Caribbean and the social and economic structures as well as the political culture of the United States. This body of work provides resources for scholars and researchers and provides instrumental strategies for use in practice by counselors/social workers, curriculum developers, and immigration analysts.*

Immigrants and Social Work: Thinking Beyond the Borders of the United States, edited by Diane Drachman, PhD, and Ana Paulino, EdD (Vol. 2, No. 1/2, 2004). *"Highly Informative . . . . The authors explain and illustrate vital concepts such as transnationalism, return migration, and circular migration. Each chapter examines changes in the United States' immigration laws in the aftermath of 9/11 and their respective impacts on the suffering of immigrant populations. Chapters on the establishment of voluntary social services in Armenia and on international social work practice are bonuses for the reader. I thank professors Drachman and Paulino for placing a 'spotlight' on a substantive area fundamental to contemporary social work practice." (Alex Gitterman, EdD, Professor of Social Work, University of Connecticut School of Social Work; Editor of* "The Legacy of William Schwartz: Group Practice as Shared Interaction")

The Health and Well-Being of Caribbean Immigrants in the United States

Annette M. Mahoney, DSW
Editor

The Health and Well-Being of Caribbean Immigrants in the United States has been co-published simultaneously as *Journal of Immigrant & Refugee Services*, Volume 2, Numbers 3/4 2004.

The Haworth Social Work Practice Press
An Imprint of The Haworth Press, Inc.

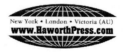

New York • London • Victoria (AU)
www.HaworthPress.com

Published by

The Haworth Social Work Practice Press, 10 Alice Street, Binghamton, NY 13904-1580 USA.

The Haworth Social Work Practice Press is an imprint of The Haworth Press, Inc., 10 Alice Street, Binghamton, NY 13904-1580 USA.

The Health and Well-Being of Caribbean Immigrants in the United States has been co-published simultaneously as *Journal of Immigrant & Refugee Services*, Volume 2, Numbers 3/4 2004.

Cover design by Lora Wiggins

Library of Congress Cataloging-in-Publication Data

The health and well-being of Caribbean immigrants in the United States / Annette M. Mahoney, editors.
     p. cm.
     "Co-published simultaneously as Journal of immigration & refugee services, volume 2, numbers 3/4, 2004."
     Includes bibliographical references and index.
     ISBN 0-7890-0442-9 (alk. paper) – ISBN 0-7890-0446-1 (pbk: alk. paper)
     1. Caribbean Americans–Social conditions. 2. Caribbean Americans–Health and hygiene I. Mahoney, Annette M. II. Journal of immigration & refugee services.
  E184 .C27H43 2004
  362.84´969729073–dc22
                                     2004012487

Indexing, Abstracting & Website/Internet Coverage

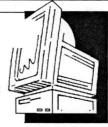

This section provides you with a list of major indexing & abstracting services. That is to say, each service began covering this periodical during the year noted in the right column. Most Websites which are listed below have indicated that they will either post, disseminate, compile, archive, cite or alert their own Website users with research-based content from this work. (This list is as current as the copyright date of this publication.)

Abstracting, Website/Indexing Coverage . . . . Year When Coverage Began

- *caredata CD: the social and community care database*
  <http://www.scie.org.uk> **2003**
- *e-psyche, LLC <http://www.e-psyche.net>* **2002**
- *Family & Society Studies Worldwide <http://www.nisc.com>* **2002**
- *Family Index Database <http://www.familyscholar.com>* **2003**
- *FINDEX <http://www.publist.com>* **2002**
- *GEO Abstracts (GEO Abstracts/GEOBASE)*
  <http://www.elsevier.nl> **2003**
- *IBZ International Bibliography of Periodical*
  Literature <http://www.saur.de> **2002**
- *Index to Periodical Articles Related to Law* **2002**
- *Internationale Bibliographie der geistes- und*
  sozialwissenschaftlichen Zeitschriftenliteratur . . . . See IBZ **1999**
- *"LABORDOC" Library–Periodicals Section*
  "Abstracts Section" **2002**
- *Peace Research Abstracts Journal* **2002**
- *Published International Literature On Traumatic Stress*
  (The PILOTS Database) <http://www.ncptsd.org> **2004**
- *Social Work Abstracts*
  <http://www.silverplatter.com/catalog/swab.htm> **2002**

(continued)

Special Bibliographic Notes related to special journal issues
(separates) and indexing/abstracting:

- indexing/abstracting services in this list will also cover material in any "separate" that is co-published simultaneously with Haworth's special thematic journal issue or DocuSerial. Indexing/abstracting usually covers material at the article/chapter level.
- monographic co-editions are intended for either non-subscribers or libraries which intend to purchase a second copy for their circulating collections.
- monographic co-editions are reported to all jobbers/wholesalers/approval plans. The source journal is listed as the "series" to assist the prevention of duplicate purchasing in the same manner utilized for books-in-series.
- to facilitate user/access services all indexing/abstracting services are encouraged to utilize the co-indexing entry note indicated at the bottom of the first page of each article/chapter/contribution.
- this is intended to assist a library user of any reference tool (whether print, electronic, online, or CD-ROM) to locate the monographic version if the library has purchased this version but not a subscription to the source journal.
- individual articles/chapters in any Haworth publication are also available through the Haworth Document Delivery Service (HDDS).

The Health and Well-Being of Caribbean Immigrants in the United States

CONTENTS

Foreword   xi
Annette M. Mahoney

Introduction: The Health and Social Well-Being
of Caribbean Immigrants in the United States   1
Annette M. Mahoney

PHYSICAL AND MENTAL HEALTH

Health, Poverty and Service Use Among Older
West Indian Women in Greater Hartford   11
Peta-Anne Baker

Disparities in Infant Mortality Rates Among
Immigrant Caribbean Groups in New York City   29
Marcia Bayne-Smith
Yvonne J. Graham
Marco A. Mason
Michelle Drossman

Confronting the Reality: An Overview of the Impact
of HIV/AIDS on the Caribbean Community   49
Mary Spooner
Carol Ann Daniel
Annette M. Mahoney

Working with Caribbean Immigrants
  After the World Trade Center Tragedy:
  A Challenge for Social Work Practice   69
    Lear Matthews

SOCIAL WELL-BEING

Caribbean Women's Migratory Journey: An Exploration of Their
  Decision-Making Process   83
    Christiana Best-Cummings
    Margery A. Gildner

Developing a Model Intervention to Prevent Abuse
  in Relationships Among Caribbean
  and Caribbean-American Youth by Partnering with Schools   103
    Kristine A. Herman

Protecting Victims of Domestic Violence
  in Caribbean Communities   117
    Mary Spooner

Social Work with West Indian Families:
  A Multilevel Approach   135
    Carol Ann Daniel

Impact of the 1996 Welfare Reform
  and Illegal Immigration Reform
  and Immigrant Responsibility Acts
  on Caribbean Immigrants   147
    Velta Clarke

Index   167

ABOUT THE EDITOR

Annette M. Mahoney, DSW, is an Assistant Professor at the Hunter College School of Social Work, City University of New York. She teaches graduate courses in Social Policy, Human Behavior, and Social Work practice with substance abusers and with victims of violence. She served as the coordinator of the part-time MSW program at Hunter College from 2001-2003. Dr. Mahoney has published articles in scholarly journals on issues related to the Caribbean immigrant population, crime and violence, and trauma and recovery. She has been active in community agencies focused on issues impacting immigrant populations, victims of violence and incarcerated women and adolescents. Additionally, she has had a long working relationship with the New York-based Caribbean Women's Health Association where she presently serves as a member of the Board of Directors. She has presented scholarly papers at various national and international conferences.

Foreword

This special collection of articles highlights a broad range of issues relating to the health and social well-being of Caribbean immigrants in the United States. The educators, researchers and community leaders who have contributed to this volume address unique challenges faced by this population. The articles are of scholarly merit, multidimensional in scope and provide comprehensive discussion of the issues, policies and interventions. This body of work provides resources for scholars and researchers in several disciplines, including social work and sociology. Persons interested in Caribbean and international affairs may also find this volume informative and enlightening.

I am grateful to the authors who have contributed to this volume. I am especially indebted to the following persons who have generously committed their time and energy to serve as reviewers of manuscripts: Janet Becker, PhD, Peggy Brown, CSW, and ABD, Irene Chung, PhD, Elizabeth Danto, PhD, Bernadette Hadden, PhD, Cynthia Johnson, CSW, and Christina Ramirez, CSW. I also wish to thank Valerie Farrell, CSW, for her generous support and assistance in the editing process and organization of this body of work.

To the Caribbean immigrants in the United States, especially those who participated in the research studies that underpin this volume–to you, I dedicate this volume.

Annette M. Mahoney
Editor

[Haworth co-indexing entry note]: "Foreword." Mahoney, Annette M. Co-published simultaneously in *Journal of Immigrant & Refugee Services* (The Haworth Social Work Practice Press, an imprint of The Haworth Press, Inc.) Vol. 2, No. 3/4, 2004, p. xv; and: *The Health and Well-Being of Caribbean Immigrants in the United States* (ed: Annette M. Mahoney) The Haworth Social Work Practice Press, an imprint of The Haworth Press, Inc., 2004, p. xi. Single or multiple copies of this article are available for a fee from The Haworth Document Delivery Service [1-800-HAWORTH, 9:00 a.m. - 5:00 p.m. (EST). E-mail address: docdelivery@haworthpress.com].

Introduction:
The Health and Social Well-Being
of Caribbean Immigrants
in the United States

Annette M. Mahoney

The health and social well-being of immigrants in the United States are best understood in terms of the social capital they bring with them, their integration into the social, economic and political context of their new society and the extent to which their distinctive characteristics promote or hinder their social mobility. This conceptualization recognizes the reciprocal processes of accommodation and adaptation as likely influences on the outcome of the immigrant's experiences. In keeping with this view, an understanding must be developed of the contributions that Caribbean immigrants make to their new communities, their progress as a group as well as the stressors that negatively impact their lives in the United States. Considerations of the life cycle are also critical in analyzing the different challenges that may emerge from one developmental stage to another. This volume attempts to paint a clear picture of how Caribbean immigrants are faring in the United States. The authors address a broad cross-section of issues related to the health and well-being of Caribbean immigrants at different stages of development and offer culturally specific prescriptive intervention models.

[Haworth co-indexing entry note]: "Introduction: The Health and Social Well-Being of Caribbean Immigrants in the United States." Mahoney, Annette M. Co-published simultaneously in *Journal of Immigrant & Refugee Services* (The Haworth Social Work Practice Press, an imprint of The Haworth Press, Inc.) Vol. 2, No. 3/4, 2004, pp. 1-9; and: *The Health and Well-Being of Caribbean Immigrants in the United States* (ed: Annette M. Mahoney) The Haworth Social Work Practice Press, an imprint of The Haworth Press, Inc., 2004, pp. 1-9. Single or multiple copies of this article are available for a fee from The Haworth Document Delivery Service [1-800-HAWORTH, 9:00 a.m. - 5:00 p.m. (EST). E-mail address: docdelivery@haworthpress.com].

CARIBBEAN PEOPLES, WHO ARE THEY?

Caribbean and West Indian are terms that are used interchangeably in reference to a group of peoples from an archipelago of islands which stretch from the tip of Florida to the coast of South America in the body of water called the Caribbean Sea. This definition usually includes some peoples from outside of that region, including Guyana in South America and segments of the population in Panama, Costa Rica and Belize, where ethnic enclaves of predominantly English-speaking Caribbean peoples reside. There is considerable ethnic and cultural heterogeneity among Caribbean peoples, however, most share the common legacy of European colonialism and African ancestry. These shared common experiences work in tandem to shape a unique Caribbean culture, a culture that extends far beyond the distinct speech patterns, food and music. Vestiges of colonialism are still evident in many of the social and political institutions within the region–in the structures of educational and legal systems and possibly in the migratory practices of Caribbean peoples.

Emigration has always been an integral component of the Caribbean experience. The search for a "better life for themselves and their children" has taken Caribbean peoples all over the globe–to countries within their own region, as well as metropolitan countries such as Britain, Canada and the United States. The United States has, however, been a favorite destination due to its burgeoning economy which promises an improved quality of life for skilled and unskilled, documented and undocumented persons who are willing to work hard in pursuit of their dreams. This movement of peoples has been significantly influenced by world economic trends, population pressure, the limited resources and opportunities available within small island states and by the prevailing immigration laws within receiving countries. The current Caribbean community comprises a significant number of persons who migrated after the enactment of the United States Immigration Reform of 1965 which allowed for admission based on job skills and on family reunification. Following this, over one million West Indians have been granted legal immigrant status, with over 600,000 of these arriving between 1981 and 1996 alone (U.S. Immigration and Naturalization Service, cited by Crowder & Tedrow, 2001). Despite the fact that the economies and social life of Caribbean countries are heavily reliant on transnational migration to the United States and other developed countries, high volumes of immigration from the region threaten a dramatic " brain drain" which will limit the ability of these nations to acquire self-sufficiency. Data cited by Waters (2000) show that small islands such as St. Kitts, Nevis and Grenada were sending 1 to 2% of their citizens to the United States every year during the 1980s. During the same period, Jamaica sent 213,805 people to the U.S.–a full 9% of its total population of 2.5 million people. Guyana, too, was sending a large proportion of its population, counted in 1984 at 775,000. With an increasing desire by developed countries, including the United States, to make their immigration laws more attractive to highly skilled foreign nationals, the Caribbean loses a significant number of its professionals, craftspeople, managers and technicians to the United States, Canada and Britain each year. The interest of capitalism in the United States is further served by the skilled and unskilled labor of immigrants from the Caribbean, large numbers of whom assume low-level jobs that offer meager salaries–jobs that native born probably would not accept. Caribbean economies, on the other hand, rely heavily on remittances from its citizens living abroad. In Jamaica, for example, private remittances to that nation during the latter half of the 1990s totaled US $3.2 Billion dollars. On an annual basis, these inflows have equaled between 9-10% of GDP. (http://www. iadb.org/mif/v2/files/grassless.doc).

Caribbean Immigrants in the United States

While pockets of Caribbean peoples can be found in virtually every state in the Union, New York has always been their favorite destination. Kasinitz (1993) notes that part of New York's attraction lies with its large numbers of earlier immigrants who have made the ethnic neighborhoods more inviting and accommodating for new immigrants as well as the wide array of institutions and services that are readily available to them. The number of Caribbean immigrants in New York has increased rapidly in the past few decades. Salvo and Ortiz (1992) note that among the 1980s cohorts of Caribbean immigrants, 45% of Jamaican immigrants live in New York, as do 49% of Trinidadians, 61% of all Barbadians and 70% of all Guyanese. Since then, there has been an even more significant growth among the population of people claiming West Indian ancestry. Waters (1999) reports a growth rate from 172,192 in 1980 to 391,744 in 1990, an increase of 127.5%. Recent estimates put their numbers at roughly 600,000, which constitutes almost one-third of New York's black population (Rogers, 2001). These numbers are regarded by some as conservative because peoples who are undocumented are likely to be excluded from the count.

The median household incomes of Caribbean immigrants in New York are higher than most other immigrant groups, as well as for African Americans, notes Kasinitz (2001). Further, he argues that their labor force participation is strikingly high, particularly for women, and their high household incomes are partially explained by the fact that nearly a quarter of West-Indian households report three or more wage earners. These findings support the argument that segments of the Caribbean American population are making great strides in education, income, and other indicators of social mobility. Many of these immigrants have improved their social and political standing and are poised to realize the American dream. On the other hand, a growing segment of the immigrant Caribbean population faces a range of challenges in measures of education, income and other indices of social well-being. Many of them have few marketable skills and occupy niches within the society that increase their vulnerability to social and economic marginalization. Studies have consistently shown that people in lower strata of income, education, and occupation are about two to three times more likely than those in the highest strata to have mental disorders (Holzer et al., 1986; Reiger et al., 1993; Muntaner et al., 1998). They are also more likely to have higher levels of psychological distress (Eaton & Muntaner, 1999; cited in the U.S. Surgeon General's Report, 1999) and overall poor health (Yen & Syme, 1999). Further, regardless of the differences in the social and economic location of Caribbean immigrants, there is a general belief that they are at increased risk for encountering various types of structural barriers due to their racial and cultural characteristics. Both Crowder and Tedrow (2001) and Kasinitz (1993) have noted that Caribbean immigrants face the prospect of assimilating into the country's most stigmatized racial groups. They argue further that in response to this fate there is a strong motivation among Caribbean immigrants to maintain their ethnic distinctiveness. However, this does not insulate them from the disparaging stereotypes associated with their phenotypic characteristics and the anti-immigrant sentiments that pervade parts of the American society.

RACE, POVERTY AND MARGINAL NEIGHBORHOODS

The American experience, despite its undisputed benefits and vast opportunities, is likely to take a toll on the health and well-being of a vast number of Caribbean children and their families. Having come from societies where people of African ancestry are in the majority, the patterns of racial and ethnic divisions that many of them encounter within the United States do not escape their attention. The stark reality of being relegated to "communities of color" includes a further realization that their new communities are notorious for characteristics which make them poor indicators of success. In their book, American Apartheid, Douglas Massey and Nancy Denton describe the segregation indices for black Americans in many U.S. cities, including New York City, as constituting hyper segregation–indeed an American form of the racial separation of apartheid (cited by Waters, 2001, p. 243). In New York City, Caribbean communities are among the most racially segregated. Attendance information from the NYC Board of Education (1999-2000) shows that school district #17 in Brooklyn, with its high concentration of Caribbean immigrants in Crown Heights, Flatbush and East Flatbush, had 87% black students; 9.4% Hispanic; 1.9% Asian and a 0.8% student population of European background. In describing the effects of residential segregation, Massey and Denton quoted above, argue that active discrimination and institutional racism lead to declining city services and declining private investment in residentially segregated neighborhoods.

Noting that the high school system in New York is built around neighborhoods, Waters (2001) estimates that approximately half of the West Indian youth population within urban and suburban areas attend schools that are in dire condition. She found that many of these schools were plagued by low academic achievement, high levels of violence, chaos, and high drop-out rates. Additionally, many of the neighborhood communities face daunting problems of poverty, drug-use, and various other indicators of poor health. Children and adolescents who reside in these socially disorganized areas face an increased risk for academic failure, delinquency and other forms of maladaptive behavior. It is the blocked mobility inherent in the combination of structural racism, racially segregated and disinvested neighborhoods, that Waters believes give rise to cultural and psychological responses described as disinvestments and oppositional identity, whereby children, in an effort to protect themselves from indignities, may disinvest, especially from school, redefining social norms and behaviors such as success in school, speaking standard English, and so forth as oppositional to their core identities. Further, Williams and Williams-Morris (2000) argue that racism and discrimination are stressful events that can directly lead to psychological and physiological changes affecting mental health.

HEALTH AND MENTAL HEALTH OF CARIBBEAN IMMIGRANTS

Caribbean immigrants are apt to face various health and mental health challenges due in part to their immigrant status, being members of an ethnic or racial minority group, their overall lower socioeconomic status, and their distinct cultural and social attitudes. An escalating problem faced by Caribbean immigrants concerns the health and well-being of its elderly populations, many of whom were uprooted from their societies to join their children and other family members here in the United States. Driven by the fear of crime in some of their native countries and the weakening ties between themselves and their homelands, other elderly Caribbean immigrants are now spending their retirement years in cities and towns across America instead of returning to their homelands as their earlier cohorts did. Also of concern is the diminished support of the extended family, as well as the unfamiliar models of care that they may encounter. Other concerns for the health of elderly Caribbean immigrants pertain to their social and economic condition. This is especially critical given the fact that large numbers of them worked in sectors of the American economy which offered meager incomes and limited, if any, retirement and health benefits.

Peta-Anne Baker pays attention to the vulnerability of elderly immigrants in a cross-sectional exploratory study of aging in the West Indian migrant community of Greater Hartford, Connecticut. She offers much insight into the state of the health and mental health of older West Indians. Her findings reveal positive self-reports of health and few limiting or disabling conditions within this population. However, she found substantial income inequality and limited use of services, especially among women who were most likely to require such services. She offers a community-based intervention strategy for working with this population.

Baker's study is followed by that of *Marcia Bayne-Smith, Yvonne Graham, Marco Mason* and *Michelle Drossman* whose paper examines infant mortality rates (IMR) among Caribbean immigrants and other ethnic groups in NYC. Their findings show that infant mortality rates (IMR) among Caribbean immigrants rank among the highest in New York City. The authors discuss causative and etiological factors that contribute to the high rates of IMR and provide readers with clearly delineated policy approaches aimed at addressing the disparities.

In their paper, *Confronting the Reality: An Overview of the Impact of HIV/AIDS on the Caribbean Community, Mary Spooner, Carol Ann Daniel* and *Annette Mahoney* highlight the serious threat that this disease now presents to the Caribbean population at home (in the Caribbean) and here in the United States. The barriers created by sociocultural, attitudinal and gender inequities are explored, highlighting the need for culturally specific interventions.

The emotional stress which often accompanies migration can be exacerbated when immigrants find themselves in a state of vulnerability as the host society responds to social crises. *Lear Matthews* examines the impact of the World Trade Center tragedy on Caribbean immigrants, arguing that their mental health and social well-being are at risk because of their marginality. He challenges human service workers to reassess their intervention with this population, taking into account the changing psychosocial functioning of this population as well as the changing immigration laws.

THE SOCIAL WELL-BEING OF CARIBBEAN IMMIGRANTS

Caribbean immigrants who leave their home countries to seek their fortunes in the United States make deliberate choices about the process of resettlement.

Christiana Best-Cummings and *Margery Gildner* explore the sometimes painful and ambivalent decision-making processes for many Caribbean women who migrate to the United States. Using case examples, the authors provide practitioners with an understanding of the migration process, the challenges of economic survival, leaving loved ones and children behind, parenting children from a distance, loneliness and adjusting to a new environment while supporting themselves and family members at home. The study offers a unique glimpse into the challenges faced by many immigrant Caribbean women, providing practitioners with valuable resources for future work with this population.

Acknowledging the growing trend of violence in relationships among young people, *Kristine Herman's* article, *Developing a Model Intervention to Prevent Abuse in Relationships Among Caribbean and Caribbean-American Youth by Partnering with Schools*, proposes a culturally specific model intervention for Caribbean youths. By partnering with community schools, she recognizes the significant role that schools play in the lives of immigrant children and adolescents. She offers educators and other helping professionals an excellent response to the burgeoning problem of school violence.

Behaviors and attitudes of social groupings such as Caribbean immigrants are often established in the countries of origin. Hence, when immigrants move to other countries, they frequently take these behaviors and attitudes with them. In her study of domestic violence in the Caribbean island of Barbados, *Mary Spooner* found that even with legislative provisions, women seldom sought refuge in the court system. In extrapolating her findings to Caribbean women in the United States, her article, *Restraining Orders in the Caribbean Community: Protecting Victims of Domestic Violence*, raises concern that women for a host of reasons–loss of economic support, family ties, fear of deportation, misguided belief in male headship of the home and subservience to men–might continue to expose themselves to domestic violence even in the United States where the laws provide more comprehensive support for victims. The findings challenge advocates and service providers here in the United States as well as in the home countries in the Caribbean to press for more sensitive policy responses to victims of domestic violence.

Carol Ann Daniel's paper, *Social Work with West Indian Immigrants: A Multilevel Approach*, explores the psychosocial and cultural experiences of Caribbean immigrants. In her work she focuses on the social, economic and related factors that impact the needs of Caribbean immigrants and proposes a multilevel model for engaging this population. Her approach includes such activities as cultural bridging, advocacy and empowerment.

The final paper examines the impact of the 1996 Welfare Reform and Illegal Immigration Reform and Immigrant Responsibility Acts on Caribbean immigrants in the United States. The author, *Velta Clarke*, tackles the contentious provision of the IIRA which allows for the deportation of immigrants who have become entangled with the criminal justice system in the U.S. She describes the impact of this policy on small developing countries in the Caribbean and on families in the United States whose members have been deported. Using a policy analysis framework, she analyzes the right of government to regulate its borders versus the human and civil rights of immigrants.

CONCLUSION

The articles in this volume offer new findings and insight into the lives of the diverse immigrant Caribbean population in the United States. The publication is particularly timely given the unique challenges faced by Caribbean immigrants as discussed in the various articles. This publication will coincide with the almost fortieth year anniversary of the Immigration Reform Act of 1965 which opened the way for large numbers of Caribbean immigrants to enter the U.S. Caribbean immigrants have influenced and have been influenced by their new society, as other immigrant groups have. Their capacity to adapt to an environment which offers as many opportunities as it poses risks is tempered by a tradition of accommodation and compromise between the host and the receiving society. The timeliness of reexamining the complexities of this relationship and the impact on immigrant families is unprecedented. The findings and conclusions of the authors in this presentation reveal the multidimensional factors that social scientists, human service professionals and policymakers must contend with in their continuous efforts to find solutions to problems relating to the health and well-being of this growing segment of the United States population.

REFERENCES

Crowder, K., Tedrow, L. (2001). West Indians and residential landscape of New York. In: Foner, Nancy; *Islands in the City: West Indian Migration to New York.* Berkeley: University of California Press, 81-114.

Eaton, W.W., & Muntaner, C. (1999). Socioeconomic stratification and mental disorder. In: *Culture counts: The influence of culture and society on mental health, mental Illness.* U.S. Surgeon General Report, 25-44.

Foner, N. (2001). Introduction: West Indian migration to New York. In: *Islands in the City: West Indian Migration to New York.* University of California Press, 1-21.

Holzer, C., Shea, B., Swanson, J., Leaf, P., Myers, J., George, L., Weissman, M., Bednarski, P. (1986). The increased risk for specific psychiatrics among persons of low socioeconomic status. *American Journal of Social Psychiatry, 6,* 259-271.

Kasinitz, P. (1993). *Caribbean New York: Black Immigrants: The Politics of Race.* New York: Cornell, University Press.

Kasinitz, P. (2001). Invisible no more. In: *Islands in the City: West Indian Migration to New York*, University of California Press, 257-275.

Muntaner, C., Eaton, W.W., Diala, C., Kessler, R.C., & Sorlie, P.D. (1998). Social class, assets, organizational control and the prevalence of common groups of Psychiatric disorders. *Social Science and Medicine, 47,* 2043-2053.

Regier, D.A, Narrow, W.E., Rae, D.S., Manderscheild, R.W., Locke, B.Z., & Goodwin, F.K. (1993). The defacto U.S. mental and addictive disorders service system. Epidemiologic Catchment Area prospective 1-2 year prevalence rates of disorders and services. *Archives of General Psychiatry, 50,* 85-94.

Salvo, J., & Ortiz, R. (1992). *The Newest New Yorkers: An Analysis of Immigration into New York City During the 1980's.* New York City Department of Planning.

Williams, D.R. & Williams-Morris, R. (2000). Racism and mental health: The African-American experience. *Ethnicity and Health*, 5, 243-268.

Yen, I.H., & Syme, S.L. (1999). The social environment and health: A discussion of the epidemiologic literature. *Annual Review of Public Health, 20,* 287-308.

Health, Poverty and Service Use Among Older West Indian Women in Greater Hartford

Peta-Anne Baker

SUMMARY. This study brings to light the phenomenon of aging in the West Indian migrant community in the United States. It presents the results of a cross-sectional exploratory survey of 107 community-dwelling West Indian women aged 55 years and over living in the Greater Hartford region of Connecticut. The data analysis reveals positive self-reports of health and few limiting or disabling conditions. However, there is substantial income inequality, a negative relationship between age group and income and limited use of services among those women most likely to require them. The findings suggest

Peta-Anne Baker, PhD, is a lecturer in the Department of Psychology, Sociology and Social Work at the University of the West Indies, Mona Campus in Jamaica (E-mail: Petaanne.baker@uwimona.edu.jm).

[Haworth co-indexing entry note]: "Health, Poverty and Service Use Among Older West Indian Women in Greater Hartford." Baker, Peta-Anne. Co-published simultaneously in *Journal of Immigrant & Refugee Services* (The Haworth Social Work Practice Press, an imprint of The Haworth Press, Inc.) Vol. 2, No. 3/4, 2004, pp. 11-28; and: *The Health and Well-Being of Caribbean Immigrants in the United States* (ed: Annette M. Mahoney) The Haworth Social Work Practice Press, an imprint of The Haworth Press, Inc., 2004, pp. 11-28. Single or multiple copies of this article are available for a fee from The Haworth Document Delivery Service [1-800-HAWORTH, 9:00 a.m. - 5:00 p.m. (EST). E-mail address: docdelivery@haworthpress.com].

that some of the qualities which contributed to West Indians becoming the "Black success model" in the U.S. may be counterproductive for successful aging. A community-based strategy for addressing these issues is outlined. *[Article copies available for a fee from The Haworth Document Delivery Service: 1-800-HAWORTH. E-mail address: <docdelivery@haworthpress.com> Website: <http://www.HaworthPress.com> © 2004 by The Haworth Press, Inc. All rights reserved.]*

KEYWORDS. Older West Indian women, West Indian immigrants, ethnic minority aging, foreign born, service use

INTRODUCTION

In 1994, 90% of the population of older adults in the United States was of European ancestry. By 2050 this proportion is expected to decline to 80%. Meanwhile the population of older Blacks, Hispanics, Asians and Pacific Islanders and indigenous peoples will double or triple, fueled by large-scale immigration, the increased longevity of these groups and the declining fertility of the European ancestry population (U.S. Bureau of the Census, 1995).

Ethnic minority elders have higher rates of poverty and a greater dependence on Social Security and other income support programs than older Whites (Binstock, 1999). However, only a small proportion of minority elders eligible for assistance actually participate in such programs (Wray, 1991). Kart and Beckham (1976, reported in Kart, 1993) found that Black elders were overrepresented in state mental hospitals and underrepresented in homes for the aged. In fact low rates of utilization of services and differential access to the various types of services are significant features of the ethnic minority elderly population (Barresi and Stull, 1993; Binstock, 1999; Harel and Biegel, 1995).

There have been many attempts to identify the reasons for this fact. Language, physical and social isolation, agency policies and staff perceived as "outsiders" (Gelfand and Yee, 1991; Harel and Biegel, 1995), ineligibility (due to non-citizen and migrant status), and inadequate financial resources (Gelfand, 1994; Keith and Jones, 1995; Wray, 1991) are among the most frequently cited barriers.

A study by Hernandez-Gallegos, Capitman and Yee (1993) highlighted several ways, including staffing and a lack of outreach, in which the features of provider organizations created barriers to access to services by minority elders. Miller and Stull (1999) in a study of Black and White elders' perceptions of community services supported these findings, reporting that Black elders commented on the gate-keeping function of agencies and practitioners.

The West Indian population is part of a larger Caribbean group that is traditionally subsumed within the Latin American region. This region has the smallest proportion of persons aged fifty-five and over (14.1%) or sixty-five and over (6.7%) (U.S. Census Bureau, 2002a). However, a very different picture emerges when the Caribbean is disaggregated from Latin America. The ratio of older persons from the wider Caribbean is greater than that of the foreign born population as a whole. (Persons fifty-five and over are 19.6% of all foreign born and those sixty-five and over are 10.2% of this group.) The Caribbean ranks second only to the European origin population in the relative size of its older population with some 29.8% of the population being aged fifty-five years and over and 16% of the population being aged sixty-five years and over (U.S. Census Bureau, 2002b). Women also predominate in this population with Caribbean migrant women constituting 55.8% and 57.3% of persons aged fifty years and over and sixty-five years and over respectively.

It is almost impossible to determine from currently published sources the size and status of older West Indians in general and West Indian women in particular. Using the Current Population Survey 2000 estimates cited above, the West Indian ancestry population is some 1.87 million. Given the duration of the West Indian presence in the United States one can reasonably assume that the ratios for the older Caribbean population can be applied to the West Indian population. I therefore estimate that there are some 557,000 persons of West Indian ancestry aged fifty-five years and over, and a little over 310,000 West Indians aged sixty-five years and over, with close to 60% of these persons being women.

Several studies highlight the presence and agency of immigrant women, especially those from the Caribbean (Cordero-Guzman and Grosfoguel, 2000; Watkins-Owens, 2001). In the field of migration studies, women still tend to be viewed as dependents who migrate to join their male breadwinner partner. In fact, women make up just under 50% of total international migration flows and a majority of the immigrant flows to most developed countries. In the United States, for example, female immigrants have been in the majority since the 1930s (DeLaet, 1998; Zlotnik, 1995). Gordon notes that the shift in the designation of female migrants from "immigrant wives" to "immigrant women" is indicative of "more than a change in terminology. It reflects a rejection of the assumption, stated or implied, that immigrants are men and dependents are women and children" (1990, pp. 116-117). A recent study of the role of Caribbean women in supporting migration from the region to New York City demonstrates that the number of female Afro-Caribbean immigrants to the United States was already on the rise at the turn of the twentieth century (Watkins-Owens, 2001).

Like migration studies, gendered perspectives in gerontology and aging policy highlight the dominance of the "male worker model" (Steckenrider, 1998). In addition, as Novak (1997) notes, the focus of gerontology has tended to be on the older white population, although there is a growing recognition of the diversification of the older population of the United States.

There has been relatively limited attention to older migrants *qua* migrants in part due to the inadequacy of data especially for small populations (Angel and Hogan, 1992). Taeuber and Allen (1993) in their analysis of demographic trends in the United States document the significant difference in earnings and receipt of benefits of older women in general and women of color in particular. These outcomes are further negatively affected by women's gendered roles as caretakers, especially of the very young and very old. They also note that higher levels of educational attainment are associated with a more favorable health outlook. It should come as no surprise that health status when measured by functional limitation, was found to be poorest among older Black women.

We do not know if the tendency of West Indian migrant women to be better educated, translates into an enhanced health status in later life. It is tempting to assume that older immigrant women, and older West Indian women in particular, will demonstrate the same tendency towards negative outcomes found among older women in general and older women of color in particular. However, this assumption is not justified until the question is more thoroughly interrogated.

Beverly Lyons' (1997) comparative analysis of service use among native born and West Indian Blacks focuses on New York as do the majority of studies of West Indian migrants. Lyons' data is only partially disaggregated by gender and it is difficult to explore socioeconomic characteristics such as income and education. Indeed the view that West Indians have emerged as a "recognizable presence" in the United States (Vickerman, 1999), is not reflected in relation to the older members of this community. One possible cause could be the tendency in the field of social work with migrants to focus on the challenges faced by the newly arrived and their acculturation (see for example Mahoney, 2002).

The purpose of this study was to uncover the reality of aging in the West Indian community by developing a profile of older West Indian migrant women focusing on selected variables: income, poverty and health status, and benefit and service use. The location of the study in Greater Hartford, Connecticut also served to contribute to knowledge about the West Indian population outside of New York City.

RESEARCH DESIGN

This study used a cross-sectional exploratory survey design to develop a profile of community-dwelling foreign-born West Indian women aged fifty-five years and over who were resident in the Greater Hartford region of the state of Connecticut. A convenience sample was recruited from the older adult population of West Indian migrant women in the Greater Hartford area. A convenience sample approach was used because it is inexpensive and accessible, and according to Burns and Grove (1997), is useful in exploratory studies.

There was no readily available preexisting sample frame, and the costs associated with developing such a frame would have been prohibitive. Two databases served as the initial sources from which study subjects were identified. The first was a database of older residents of the Blue Hills neighborhood in the city of Hartford that was maintained by the Blue Hills Civic Association. The Blue Hills area has a high proportion of West Indian residents and has organized representation in the form of the Blue Hills Civic Association (BHCA). The Civic Association had conducted a survey of senior citizens in November 2000 and created a database with basic information including the national origin of respondents. Approximately one-third (105 persons) of those who participated in that study were reportedly West Indian. Access to this information as well as institutional support for the fieldwork for this project was provided by the BHCA.

The second database from which study participants were identified was the membership list of the West Indian Social Club of Hartford (WISC). The Club was founded in 1950 and is one of the oldest West Indian community organizations in the United States.

The names and addresses of potential participants were also obtained from the membership lists of two churches: St Justin's Catholic Church and the St. Monica's Episcopal Church, both of which have predominantly West Indian congregations. Additional subjects were recruited from surrounding neighborhoods and towns in Greater Hartford through personal visits to other churches with West Indian congregations, through contacts made with other West Indian community organizations, and through community leaders including the Deputy Mayor of the Hartford City Council who is West Indian.

Knowing the potential for bias in a convenience sample, a decision was made to compare specific data for the individuals who participated in the present study with the same data for the older female West Indian migrant population in the Greater Hartford area. A special tabulation of 1990 Census data provided a basis for evaluating the extent to which the study sample was typical of the larger population.

A profile of the population of community-dwelling foreign-born West Indian women aged fifty-five years and over living in Connecticut was created from this Census data. The variables of interest were: age, marital status, citizenship, year of arrival in the United States, number of children, income and poverty status, highest level of schooling, employment status and occupation, and mobility and self-care limitations as a means of assessing health status. These data were compiled from the "long form" version of the decennial Census survey instrument, and were obtained from the University of Minnesota Census Project–Integrated Public Use Microdata Series (IPUMS). Although the 2000 Census had been conducted while this study was underway, the data sets containing the information needed for this study were not available for public use.

Data were collected in face-to-face interviews using a structured interview schedule. Three persons, all female, assisted me with administering the questionnaire used in this study. All the members of the team, including myself, are West Indian by birth or ancestry. I expected that this shared gender and ethnic background would increase the acceptance of the interviewers by study participants. In addition to the data collected by this means, I lived in the community for two years, during which I was a participant observer in the life of the West Indian community.

DEMOGRAPHIC AND SOCIOECONOMIC CHARACTERISTICS

One-hundred and seven women from ten countries in the English-speaking Caribbean living in the Greater Hartford region of Connecticut participated in the study. Forty-four women (41.1%) were in the fifty-five to sixty-four age group, forty-eight (44.9%) were aged sixty-five to seventy-four years and fifteen (14%) were seventy-five years of age or older. Sixty-six women (61.7%) lived in shared households (i.e. with other adult kin and with or without spouses and minor children) and forty-one women (38.3%) lived in separate households (alone or with spouses and minor children only). Twenty women (18.7%) lived alone. A substantial majority (82.2%) of the respondents were naturalized citizens.

Table 1 summarizes the demographic and socioeconomic characteristics of the sample and compares it with data on the foreign born female West Indian population aged fifty-five years and over in Connecticut extracted from the 1990 Census. There are several notable similarities and differences. The mean age of the study sample is somewhat older than that reported in the Census data and there is substantial divergence in the estimates of the proportion of the population that is married. Of interest is the absence in the Census data of persons in the Executive and Managerial occupational groups, and the very small percentage of persons in the Professional occupational group in the Census data. Not only is this different from the characteristics of the study sample,

TABLE 1. Demographic and Socioeconomic Characteristics of Study Sample and Female Foreign Born West Indian Migrant Population Aged 55+ in Connecticut (Percentages Unless Otherwise Stated)

CHARACTERISTIC	STUDY SAMPLE (N = 107)	CT - 1990 IPUMS[1] (N = 1674)
AGE (in years)		
1 M	67.2	63.9
2 SD	8.4	8.43
3 Range	45.0	35.0
MARITAL STATUS		
1 Currently married, spouse resident	44.9	29.8
2 Currently married, non-resident spouse	4.7	8.7
3 Separated or divorced	18.7	21.9
4 Widowed	21.5	25.6
5 Never married/not cohabiting	10.3	14.0
TOTAL NO. OF CHILDREN	3-4 (mode)	3.75 (mean)
HIGHEST LEVEL OF SCHOOLING[2]		
1 Elementary or less	23.4	31.4
2 Did not finish high school	6.5	26.1
3 Finished high school	17.8	32.1
4 Technical or vocational training	37.4	n.a.
5 College or university	15.0	10.3
EMPLOYMENT STATUS		
1 Employed (incl. self employed)	32.7	48.8
2 Retired, returned to work	12.1	n.a.
3 Not employed, available	6.5	4.5
4 Retired, no longer working	45.8	46.7
5 Never worked in U.S.	2.8	n.a.
OCCUPATION (current or last worked)		
1 Executive/Managerial	5.8	0
2 Professional	15.5	2.5
3 Service	60.0	72.8
- Nurses aide and other health care support	(30.1)	(34.5)
- Private household	(9.7)	(8.3)
4 Sales and office	11.7	14.6
5 Self-employed	4.9	0
6 Other	1.9	9.9
ANNUAL INCOME ($) (Quintiles)		
1 20	9600	2592
2 40	15600	6996
3 60	20400	15000
4 80	20400	28000
HOME OWNERSHIP		
1 Owns (separately or with spouse)	54.7	55.7
2 Rents	9.4[3]	41.7

Notes: (1) Steven Ruggles and Matthew Sobek et al. *Integrated Public Use Microdata Series: Version 2.0,* Minneapolis: Historical Census Projects, University of Minnesota, 1997.
(2) Data for highest level of schooling are not directly comparable due to differences in school systems (Caribbean/U.S.).
(3) Only counts cases where homeowner is an unrelated person. Some respondents living in houses owned by adult children or other family members reported paying rent.

but it is at variance with other data (using Census data from an alternate source) profiling West Indian migrant women (Model, 2001).

The relatively high proportion of persons in these occupational groupings, as well as their higher levels of education compared to other immigrant groups, another feature not supported by this Census data set, are considered hallmarks of the West Indian immigrant population in the United States. These are two of the characteristics associated with the idea of West Indian immigrants representing a model of "Black success" in the U.S. In this regard, the occupational characteristics of the study sample could be considered to be more "typical" of the West Indian population.

The data describing the study sample and the Census data both highlight the preponderance of women engaged in service occupations, especially in health care support activities and private household employment. Close to 50% of both groups are still active members of the labor force (including several who have retired but are still working), and more than 50% of both groups own their own homes.

Notwithstanding this positive economic picture, the data for the study sample and from the Census point to high levels of income poverty, with between 20% and 40% of participants being at or below the poverty level, and possibly more than 50% being in an economically vulnerable position (defined as being at 150% of the official poverty threshold for this age group). The examination of this and subsequent data also confirms the existence of substantial income inequality within this group.

INCOME, HEALTH AND AGE

The analysis of the income of the study sample affords additional insight into the women's economic status. Some 23% of the group has an annual income of less than $10,000 while only an estimated 2% or 3% receive more than $30,000 annually. There were a limited number of notable cases of professional women eligible for retirement who were still in the labor force and living on joint current incomes in the region of $60,000 per year, while they put aside private pension funds for the day of their actual retirement.

The cross-tabulation of these variables in Table 2 highlights this income inequality with approximately one-third of the two older age groups having the lowest incomes. The data reveal a statistically significant negative correlation between income and age group.

A similar picture emerges when data on the poverty status of both the study sample and the 1990 Census data are examined. Table 3 provides a profile of

TABLE 2. Cross-Tabulations of Monthly Income of Study Sample by Age Group

	55 - 64 YEARS	65 - 74 YEARS	75 YEARS & OVER
APPROX. MONTHLY INCOME ($) [1]	(N = 43)	(N = 46)	(N = 14)
≤ 800	11.7	30.4	35.6
1000 - 1200	7.0	26.1	7.1
1300 - 1500	9.3	17.4	35.7
≥ 1700	72.1	26.1	21.4

Notes:
(1) Gamma -.487; p < .001

TABLE 3. Poverty Status by Age Group–Study Sample[1] and 1990 Census[2]

	55-64 years		65-74 years		75 years & over	
	Study sample	1990 Census	Study sample	1990 Census	Study sample	1990 Census
At or below poverty	11.7	8.7	30.4	17.8	35.7	51.3
Economically vulnerable[a]	18.7	11.8	56.5	40.6	42.8	51.3
Not in poverty	81.3	88.2	43.5	59.4	57.2	48.7

Notes:
(1) Gamma-.495; p < .001
(2) Gamma-.398; p < .001
(a) Economic vulnerability = persons at or below 150% of the official poverty threshold.

the poverty status of older West Indian women using data from these two sources.

A negative correlation was found between poverty status and age group in both sets of data. The proportion of economically vulnerable women in the two oldest groups is noteworthy. Overall, both data sources indicated that close to 40% of all older West Indian women are in an economically vulnerable position.

A much better picture emerges from the profile of the women's health status. Data on the existence of conditions that limit or prevent the target group from performing self-care or other routine activities are presented in Table 4. The age group to which the participants belong was found to have a statistically significant positive relationship to the presence or absence of limiting or disabling conditions.

This does not mean, however, that those women in the older age groups were automatically in poorer health than their younger counterparts. Table 5

TABLE 4. Health Status by Age Group–Study Sample[1] and 1990 Census[2]

	55-64 years		65-74 years		75 years & over			
	Study sample	1990 Census	Study sample	1990 Census	Study sample	1990 Census		
No limiting or disabling condition	79.5	83.9	64.6	46.5	40.0	55.4		
At least 1 limiting or disabling condition	20.5	16.1	35.4	53.5	60.0	44.6		

Notes:
(1) Gamma .458; p < .01
(2) Gamma .549; p < .001

presents further details about the health status of the West Indian women who participated in the study. In particular, it compares and contrasts the women's self-evaluation of their health with their response to questions concerning the presence of limiting or disabling conditions which were compiled into a health status index.

More than 50% of women aged fifty-five to sixty-four years, close to that number of women in the sixty-five to seventy-four age group and more than 30% of the women in the oldest age group rated their health as excellent or very good. No statistically significant link was found between age group and self-reported health. Of interest is the fact that none of the women in the seventy-five and over age group rated their health as poor, although a small percentage (13%) reported substantial limitations and disabilities. On the other hand, several of those in the younger age groups felt themselves to be in fair health despite the absence of many limiting or disabling conditions.

A significant link between age group and health status was found when a less subjective self-report measure was used, that is, the identification of the existence of limitations of the ability to perform basic activities of daily living. However, even with this measure it appeared that the relatively high incidence of economic vulnerability discussed above, did not translate into perceptions or experiences of ill health.

BENEFITS AND SERVICE USE

The profile of this group of older West Indian women in Greater Hartford was completed by an examination of their receipt of cash benefits and use of services. This part of the analysis focused on those women who were most

TABLE 5. Cross Tabulations for Self-Reported Health, Limitations and Disability by Age Group (in Percentages)

	55 - 64 YEARS	65 - 74 YEARS	75 YEARS & OVER
SELF-REPORTED HEALTH	(N = 44)	(N = 47)	(N = 15)
Excellent	20.5	14.9	6.7
Very Good	38.6	34.0	26.7
Good	18.2	29.8	46.7
Fair	20.5	17.0	20.0
Poor	2.3	4.3	-
HEALTH STATUS INDEX[1,2]		(N = 48)	
None	79.5	64.6	40.0
1	13.6	18.8	13.3
2	2.3	14.6	20.0
3	-	2.1	13.3
4	4.5	-	6.7
5	-	-	6.7

Notes:
(1) Number of categories of limiting or disabling conditions
(2) Gamma .456; p < .01

likely to need the selected benefits and services, women aged sixty-five years and over, who were living at or below poverty, who were in an economically vulnerable position (at or below 150% of the poverty line), who reported that they were in fair or poor health or who had three or more limiting or disabling conditions.

Table 6 presents the frequencies for the main sources of income for women in the first three groups listed. The majority of women in all categories relied heavily on social security income. The poorest women in the age group sixty-five years and over were least likely to be receiving social security or a pension from private sources. They were more likely to have wages or salaries as a main source of income, and were also most likely to be receiving Supplemental Security Income or some other form of public assistance. A little more than a quarter of women sixty-five and over who were at or below the poverty line were not responsible for meeting their own expenses. Very few women in any of the three groups relied on spouses or children for financial support.

Table 7 reports the benefits and services received or used by women aged sixty-five years and over who were at or below the poverty line, in fair or poor health or with three or more limiting or disabling health conditions. Medicare coverage appeared to be fairly extensive among women aged sixty-five years and over, except among the poorest women, with 55.6% of those in this group receiving this benefit. In only one instance, poor women receiving SSI or

TABLE 6. Main Income Sources[1] for Women 65 Years and Over–Total, at or Below Poverty or Economically Vulnerable (in Percentages)

INCOME SOURCE	All women aged 65+ (N = 58)	Women 65+ at or below poverty (N = 24)	Women 65+ economically vulnerable (N = 40)
Social security	79.3	52.6	71.0
Private pension	46.6	15.8	32.2
Wages/salary	13.8	15.8	12.9
Spouse	1.7	-	3.2
Child	3.4	5.3	3.2
Rent/business	6.9	5.3	6.5
Interest	3.4	-	6.5
SSI/other public assistance	8.6	21.1	12.9
Not responsible for own expenses	8.6	26.3	16.1

Note:
(1) Totals exceed 100%–Women were asked to state the two main sources of income

SSDI, did the proportion of women receiving a benefit exceed 25% percent and in most instances the proportion did not exceed 10%.

The participants in the study who did not use any of the services listed or used them infrequently were asked why this was so. Table 8 sets out their responses. Of interest is the finding that except for the poorest women, 50% or more of the participants stated that they did not feel they needed these services.

Between 15% and 25% of all four groups felt or had been told that they did not qualify for services that they did attempt to obtain. In several instances, the women reported that owning their own homes–even if they were having difficulty maintaining them–proved to be a major obstacle to accessing services. Several women, close to a quarter of the poorest, had no knowledge of the services listed and of whether they were eligible to use them. A not insubstantial proportion of women reported having had a bad prior experience with service providers which made them reluctant to seek services.

The problematic situation regarding service use was reinforced in conversations with community leaders, other West Indian residents and some service providers themselves. There was a strongly held view that attending to the need of older persons was a family concern. In fact, we quickly learnt that family members sometimes needed reassurance about the purpose of the study, as

TABLE 7. Benefit and Service Use for R Aged 65+ and At or Below Poverty Level, in Fair or Poor Health, or with 3 or More Limiting or Disabling Conditions (in Percentages)

Benefit	All R aged 65+ (N = 58)	R 65+ at or below poverty (N = 19)	R 65+ in fair or poor health (N = 13)	R 65+ with 3 or more limiting/dis- abling conditions (N = 5)
Medicare	75.4	55.6	91.7	100.0
Medicaid	5.3	5.6	8.3	25.0
SSI/SSDI	19.3	27.8	16.7	-
Food stamps	3.5	11.1	-	-
Housing subsidy	1.8	5.6	-	25.0
State supplement	1.8	5.6	-	-
Home health aide	5.4	-	8.3	25.0
Meals on Wheels	3.6	5.6	8.3	-
Meals at Senior Center	10.6	5.6	16.7	-
Nursing/convalescent home	-	-	-	-
Nurses aide/personal care attendant	1.8	5.6	8.3	-
Dial-a-Ride	10.9	17.6	16.7	25.0
Adult day care	3.6	5.6	-	25.0
Senior center	16.1	11.1	16.7	-

the interviews were occasionally seen as an evaluation of how well they were attending to the needs of their older family members. Many participants as well as members of the wider community, viewed the main service providers with suspicion, and their lack of familiarity with agency procedures resulted in these being experienced as intrusive and sometimes offensive. More than one respondent was indignant at the suggestion that she would have to relinquish the house she had worked so hard to obtain in order to qualify for certain types of assistance.

Respondents who needed help had few avenues through which to seek assistance. Although the West Indian community in Hartford had achieved a measure of visibility and influence, this was exercised primarily around cultural questions. Some groups, for example the churches, and the West Indian Social Club, provided occasional assistance to members in need. However, in the main the community lacked knowledge and expertise about the social service system, particularly as it related to services for older persons. In addition, it was found that the community itself had a relatively limited appreciation of the emergence of aging as an issue in need of collective/public intervention.

TABLE 8. Reasons for Not Using Services–Respondents Aged 65+, At or Below Poverty Level, in Fair or Poor Health or With 3 or More Limiting or Disabling Conditions (in Percentages)

Reason	All R aged 65+ (N = 58)	R 65+ at or below poverty (N = 19)	R 65+ in fair or poor health (N = 13)	R 65+ with 3 or more limiting/disabling conditions (N = 5)
No need	64.8	29.4	54.5	50.0
No knowledge	11.1	23.5	9.1	-
Not qualified	14.8	23.5	18.2	25.0
Bad prior experience	9.3	23.5	18.2	25.0

CONCLUSION AND IMPLICATIONS

This exploratory study has sought to bring to light the emergence of aging in the West Indian migrant community as a phenomenon requiring systematic attention. Although the comparison with Census data reveals that the study sample shares some similarities with the population as a whole, the results of the survey cannot be truly generalized to the population of older West Indian migrant women in Connecticut. The results do, however, illustrate the need for further research which, for example, compares the situation of older women in the main geographic regions in which the West Indian population is concentrated (New York, Florida, New Jersey and Connecticut). In addition, a consistent gendered perspective also calls for research on the status of older West Indian men.

Gibson and Stoller (1998) have recommended a shift in paradigm to ensure the continued effectiveness of applied gerontology. They urge that rather than focus only on majority-minority comparisons, attention also needs to be paid to within-group variations. In fact one could argue that in the case of West Indian elders, there are two majorities: the dominant white majority and the native born Black majority.

In addition to these within-group comparisons, there is a need to engage in between-group analyses, using both race/ethnicity, i.e., comparing native born African-American elders with West Indian elders, and migrant status (comparing older foreign born West Indians with other older migrants) as the major distinguishing variables.

The data on the degree of income inequality and economic vulnerability among this segment of the older West Indian population provide another lens through which to examine the accomplishments of the West Indian migrant population in the United States. It suggests that the "Black success model" may have been constructed at a price. The study also points to the need to examine in further detail the impact of cultural values, such as the popular perception that aging is a "family affair," as well as the impact of policy changes in the welfare and immigration fields on the use of public services by those older West Indians who need them.

Changes in both immigration and welfare policy have affected migrant elders who have been in the country for some time. Some of the more draconian aspects of the Personal Responsibility and Work Opportunity Reconciliation Act (PRWORA) which would have denied legal migrants who were not citizens access to certain benefits have been eliminated. However, Urban Institute policy analysts Fix and Passel (1999) point to what they call the "chilling effect" of the several pieces of welfare and immigration reform legislation passed in the mid-1990s. They do note that no statistically significant changes in welfare use by elderly migrants were observed in the period immediately following the passage of the PRWORA. However, they also point to the fact that a lack of understanding of the changes in the law appear to have discouraged some migrants from using needed services. These findings and the results and observations of the current study make a clear case for extensive public education in the West Indian community.

A second paper (Fix and Zimmerman, 1999) discusses a similar response in "mixed-status families" where some members of the household are citizens and others are not. In this case the concerns were in relation to more stringent requirements for sponsoring family members, an increased risk of deportation or refusal of reentry if found to have become a "public charge." Given the surge in immigration from the West Indies that has occurred since 1990 (U.S. Census Bureau, 2002c), and the significant role played by older West Indian women in facilitating the entry of new migrants (Brown, 1997; Olwig, 2001; Watkins-Owens, 2001), these are real issues for the community.

Finally, any review of the development of aging policy in the United States reveals how fundamentally political a process it is (Rich and Baum, 1984; Steckenrider and Parrott, 1998; Villa, 1998). In the pluralistic competitive political environment it is those who are "visible and organized" (Ron Hill, Executive Director, Western Reserve Area Agency on Aging, personal communication, June 14, 2000) who receive attention and resources. Haitian and Hispanic groups in both New York City and Florida have raised the issue of the needs of their elderly populations in ways that Anglo Caribbeans have yet to do.

In this regard, aging is like gender and race. There is a need for a degree of consciousness raising and mobilization within the West Indian community itself. As Binstock (1999) observes, the mainstream aging membership organizations like the American Association of Retired Persons have little impetus to take up the concerns of ethnic minority elders. For minority communities such as the West Indian community, the personal or private must become political and public.

With respect to aging policy, it is worth noting Kramer and Barker's comment that smaller ethnic groups (like West Indians) receive less attention because federally mandated targeting only specifies four groups (Hispanics, Blacks, Native Americans/Native Alaskans, Asians/Pacific Islanders). They also observe that groups that lack an established local political power base are more likely to be neglected (Kramer and Barker, 1991:128). Therefore, while short- and medium-term interventions such as making services more comprehensible and accessible to West Indian migrant elders are obviously important, there is a longer-term challenge to be confronted, that of strengthening and expanding the political influence of the West Indian community so that it, too, can have its say on issues such as policies affecting the older members of the community.

REFERENCES

Angel, J. L. & Hogan, D. P. (1992). The demography of minority aging populations. *Journal of Family History, 17(1)*, 95–115.

Barresi, C. M. & Stull, D. E. (1993). Ethnicity and long-term care: An overview. In C. M. Barresi & D. E. Stull (Eds.), *Ethnic elderly and long-term care* (pp. 3–21). New York: Springer.

Binstock, R. H. (1999). Public policies and minority elders. In M. L. Wykle & A. B. Ford (Eds.), *Serving minority elders in the 21st century* (pp. 5–24). New York: Springer.

Brown, D. A. (1997). Workforce losses and return migration to the Caribbean: A case study of Jamaican nurses. In P. Pessar (Ed.), *Caribbean circuits: New directions in the study of Caribbean migration* (pp. 197–224). New York: Center for Migration Studies.

Burns, N. & Grove, S. (1997). *The practice of nursing research: Conduct, critique and utilization*. London: WB Saunders.

Campbell Gibson, R. & Stoller, E. P. (1998). Applied gerontology and minority aging: A millennial goal. *Journal of Applied Gerontology, 17(2)*, 124–128.

Cordero-Guzman, H. & Grosfoguel, R. (2000). The demographics and socio-economic characteristics of post-1965 immigrants to New York City: A comparative analysis by national origin. *International Migration, 38(4)*, 41–77.

DeLaet, D. L. (1998). The invisibility of women in scholarship on international migration. In G. A. Kelson & D. L. DeLaet (Eds.), *Gender and immigration* (pp. 1–17). Washington Square, NY: New York University Press.

Fix, M. & Passel, J. S. (1999, March). *Trends in noncitizens' and citizens' use of public benefits following welfare reform: 1994-1997.* Washington, DC: The Urban Institute. Retrieved 7/18/00 from http://www.urban.org/immig/trends.html.

Fix, M. & Zimmerman, W. (1999, June). *All under one roof: Mixed status families in an era of reform.* Washington, DC: The Urban Institute. Retrieved 7/18/00 from http://www.urban.org/immig/all_under.html

Gelfand, D. E. & Yee, B.W.K. (1991). Trends and forces: Influence of immigration, migration, and acculturation on the fabric of aging in America. *Generations, Fall/Winter*, (pp. 7–10).

Gelfand, D. E. (1994). *Aging and ethnicity: Knowledge and services.* New York: Springer.

Gordon, M. H. (1990). Dependents or independent workers? The status of Caribbean immigrant women in the United States. In R. W. Palmer (Ed.), *In search of a better life: Perspectives on migration from the Caribbean* (pp. 115–137). New York: Praeger.

Harel, Z. & Biegel, D. (1995). Aging, ethnicity, and mental health services: Social work perspectives on need and use. In D. K. Padgett (Ed.), *Handbook on ethnicity, aging, and mental health* (pp. 217–241). Westport, CT: Greenwood Press.

He, Wan (2002). *The older foreign-born population in the United States: 2000.* U.S. Census Bureau, Current Population Reports, Series P23-211. Washington, DC, 2002: U.S. Government Printing Office.

Hernandez-Gallegos, W., Capitman, J. & Yee, D. L. (1993). Conceptual understanding of long-term service use by elders of color. In C. M. Barresi & D. E. Stull (Eds.), *Ethnic elderly and long-term care* (pp. 204–220). New York: Springer.

Kart, C. S. (1993). Community-based, non-institutional long-term care service utilization by aged blacks: Facts and issues. In C. M. Barresi & D. E. Stull (Eds.), *Ethnic elderly and long-term care* (pp. 23–246). New York: Springer.

Keith, V. M & Jones, W. (1995). Determinants of health services utilization among the black and white elderly. In M. D. Feit & S. F. Battle (Eds.), *Health and social policy* (pp. 39–54). Binghamton, NY: The Haworth Press, Inc.

Kramer, B. J. & Barker, J. C. (1991). Ethnic diversity in aging and aging services in the U.S.: Introduction. *Journal of Cross-Cultural Gerontology, 6(2)*, 127–133.

Lyons, B. P. (1997). *Sociological differences between American-born and West Indian-born elderly Blacks: A comparative study of health and social service use.* New York: Garland Publishers.

Mahoney, A. (2002). Newly arrived West Indian adolescents: A call for a cohesive social welfare response to their adjustment needs. *Journal of Immigrant & Refugee Services, 1 (1)*, 33-48.

Miller, B. & Stull, D. (1999). Perceptions of community services by African American and White older persons. In C. M. Barresi & D. E. Stull (Eds.), *Ethnic elderly and long-term care* (pp. 267–286). New York: Springer.

Model, S. (2001). Where New York West Indians work. In N. Foner (Ed.), *Islands in the city: West Indian migration to New York* (pp. 52–80). Berkeley, CA: University of California Press.

Novak, M.W. (1997). *Issues in aging: An introduction to gerontology.* New York: Longman.

Olwig, K. F. (2001). New York as a locality in a global family network. In N. Foner (Ed.), *Islands in the city: West Indian migration to New York* (pp. 142–160). Berkeley, CA: University of California Press.

Rich, B. M. & Baum, M. (1984). *The aging–a guide to public policy.* Pittsburgh, PA: University of Pittsburgh Press.

Ruggles, S. & Sobek, M. et al. (1997). *Integrated Public Use Microdata Series: Version 2.0.* Minneapolis: Historical Census Projects, University of Minnesota. http://www.ipums.umn.edu

Steckenrider, J. S. & Parrott, T. M. (1998). Aging as a female phenomenon: The plight of older women. *New directions in old age policies* (pp. 235–260). Buffalo, NY: State University of New York Press.

Taeuber, C. M. & Allen, J. (1993). Women in our aging society: The demographic outlook. In J. Allen & A. Pifer (Eds.), *Women on the front lines: Meeting the challenge of an aging America* (pp. 11–46). Washington, DC: The Urban Institute Press.

U.S. Bureau of the Census (1995). *Sixty-five plus in the United States.* Statistical brief SB/95-8. Issued May 1995. U.S. Department of Commerce, Economic and Statistics Administration, Bureau of the Census.

U.S. Census Bureau (2002a). *Foreign-Born population by sex, age, and world region of birth: March 2002.* Table 3.1. Current Population Survey. Ethnic and Hispanic Statistics Branch, Population Division. Internet Release date: March 10, 2003.

U.S. Census Bureau (2002b). *Foreign-Born population by sex, age, and region of birth: March 2002.* Table 4.1. Current Population Survey, Ethnic and Hispanic Statistics Branch, Population Division. Last updated–9/24/02. [On-line]

U.S. Census Bureau (2002c). Statistical Abstract of the United States: 2002. Section 1–Population. [On-line]

Vickerman, M. (1999). *Crosscurrents: West Indian immigrants and race* (pp. 59–89). New York: Oxford University Press.

Villa, V. M. (1998). Aging policy and the experience of older minorities. In J. S Steckenrider & T. M. Parrott (Eds.), *New directions in old-age policies* (pp. 211–233). Albany, NY: State University of New York Press.

Watkins-Owens, I. (2001). Early-twentieth-century Caribbean women: Migration and social networks in New York City. In N. Foner (Ed.), *Islands in the city: West Indian migration to New York* (pp. 25–51). Berkeley, CA: University of California Press.

Wray, L. A. (1991). Public policy implications of an ethnically diverse elderly population. *Journal of Cross-Cultural Gerontology, 6(2),* 243–257.

Zlotnik, H. (1995). The south-to-north migration of women. *International Migration Review, 29(1),* 229–254.

Disparities in Infant Mortality Rates Among Immigrant Caribbean Groups in New York City

Marcia Bayne-Smith
Yvonne J. Graham
Marco A. Mason
Michelle Drossman

SUMMARY. This study examined infant mortality rates (IMR) in New York City (NYC) to identify those groups reporting higher IMR concentrations in recent years and to determine what factors and explanations are associated with this new trend.

Analysis of data from NYC Department of Health (DOH) identified infant mortality patterns throughout the City by both maternal birthplace and NYC Health Districts. In addition, infant mortality rates for those NYC populations with the highest concentrations were compared to the most recently available IMR data from their countries of origin. Focus group sessions were conducted with women in the identified groups in

Marcia Bayne-Smith, DSW, is Assistant Professor of the Urban Studies Department, Queens College–CUNY.

Yvonne J. Graham, RN, MPH, is Deputy Borough President of Brooklyn, New York City.

Marco A. Mason, DSW, is Executive Director and Michelle Drossman is Health Data Analyst of the Caribbean Women's Health Association, Inc., Brooklyn, NY.

[Haworth co-indexing entry note]: "Disparities in Infant Mortality Rates Among Immigrant Caribbean Groups in New York City." Bayne-Smith, Marcia et al. Co-published simultaneously in *Journal of Immigrant & Refugee Services* (The Haworth Social Work Practice Press, an imprint of The Haworth Press, Inc.) Vol. 2, No. 3/4, 2004, pp. 29-48; and: *The Health and Well-Being of Caribbean Immigrants in the United States* (ed: Annette M. Mahoney) The Haworth Social Work Practice Press, an imprint of The Haworth Press, Inc., 2004, pp. 29-48. Single or multiple copies of this article are available for a fee from The Haworth Document Delivery Service [1-800-HAWORTH, 9:00 a.m. - 5:00 p.m. (EST). E-mail address: docdelivery@haworthpress.com].

29

New York City in an effort to obtain their perspectives on causality and other factors associated with the new trend.

Strong patterns emerged from this study pointing to a concentration of the City's highest IMR among groups from the circum-Caribbean region. Results of focus group sessions with women in the identified population groups yielded a list of specific barriers faced by this population in the utilization of perinatal care services. In addition, the study resulted in some clearly delineated program and policy approaches that can help to address the disparities in IMR.

Myriad causative factors contribute to the high rates of IMR among Caribbean immigrant groups. Expanding the availability of both successful program models and promising practices is critical to decreasing infant mortality in immigrant communities. Specific recommendations are for the development of a strategic set of interventions designed to eliminate this most serious challenge to the health of new immigrant groups in NYC.

Any references to comparisons between data from NYC and data from the countries of origin were merely to serve as a reference point as it is not often possible to determine the level of scientific rigor applied to the collection and analysis of data external to the United States (U.S.).

Implications for social work practice with immigrant populations include the need for delivery of culturally competent services in general and for cultural sensitivity to health beliefs surrounding maternal child health issues in particular. *[Article copies available for a fee from The Haworth Document Delivery Service: 1-800-HAWORTH. E-mail address: <docdelivery@haworthpress.com> Website: <http://www.HaworthPress.com> © 2004 by The Haworth Press, Inc. All rights reserved.]*

KEYWORDS. Infant mortality rates, Caribbean region, perinatal care services, cultural barriers, service access

INTRODUCTION

Maternal and child health measures are key indicators in determining the health status of a community. In particular, infant mortality is a universally recognized indicator of the health status of any population group (Klein & Hawk, 1992; Morbidity and Mortality Weekly Report [MMWR], 1991; Singh & Yu, 1995). The international acceptance of infant mortality rates as a key health indicator is based on the recognition that infants are in many ways, the most vulnerable population group in terms of susceptibility to health adversities in their environment (Rodgers et al., 2002). In addition, infant mortality is the most reliable indicator of health, since it involves birth and death statistics which every country collects and involves "events" which, unlike the identification of various diseases, are unambiguous.

According to reports from the National Center for Health Statistics, infant mortality decreased dramatically in the United States (U.S.) throughout the course of the twentieth century with declines as high as 55% for whites and 37% for blacks in the last two decades (National Center for Health Statistics [NCHS], 1998). As a result, the U.S. has been able to recover from its embarrassingly low position as 23rd in the international IMR ranking in 1988 (Singh & Yu, 1995) to a more respectable ranking of 6th in the world as of 1999, slightly behind Norway, Australia, Canada, Sweden and Belgium (United Nations Development Programme [UNDP], 2001.

While this improvement is indeed significant for the U.S. as a whole, it has not been consistent for all population groups. For example, the 1991 US IMR of 16.5 for black infants was 2.2 times greater than the rate of 7.25 for whites (Singh & Yu, 1995). However, recent information on infant mortality from the Centers for Disease Control and Prevention (CDC) indicates that 10 years later, the 2001 IMR of 14.0 for blacks was 2.6 times greater than the rate of 5.7 for whites (CDCFastats, 2003), which suggests not only that racial disparities in health persist but that they actually continue to worsen (Henderson, 2000; NCHS, 1993). The 2001 IMR rates are a cause for serious concern because the differences went from black infants having a rate that was slightly more than twice the rate for whites in 1998 (Guyer, Freedman, Strobino & Sondik, 2000) to a rate that in 2001, was almost three times the rate for whites.

The decline in infant mortality in the U.S. is unparalleled by any other mortality reductions in the past century (MMWR, 1999), despite the fact that it has not been uniform for all groups in the population. National efforts such as the previous Healthy People 2000 and the current Healthy People 2010 were designed to address uneven health gains. Nevertheless, changes in US-IMR over time provide essential evidence of persistent disparities across racial, ethnic and class lines (McCloskey, 1999) that continue to resist elimination.

It has been well-recognized for at least three decades that the burden of mortality and morbidity in the U.S. is disproportionately borne by people of color (Bayne-Smith, 1996; U.S. Department of Health and Human Service [USDHHS], 1985). Heart disease among women provides one example in that the heart disease death rates among African American women in 1995 were 1.4 times higher than the rates for white women (Casper et al., 2000).

With regard to IMR, various explanations for the higher risk of infant mortality among racial/ethnic groups have been offered. Some studies cite higher incidence of low birth weight (LBW) and pre-term births for blacks (MMWR, 1996; McBarnette, 1996; Vohr, 1998) even when controlling for education as a proxy for socioeconomic status (Collins & Butler, 1997). Other studies suggest that sudden infant death syndrome (SIDS) has played a role in higher IMRs among American Indian and Alaska Natives (Kaufman & Joseph-Fox, 1996) and LBW has been identified as contributing to high IMR in Latinos/Hispanics (MMWR, 1999) and Asians/Pacific Islanders as well (Le, Kiely & Schoendorf, 1996). In spite of extensive research on birth outcomes of the four major population groups of color, the literature offers no explanations for the current glaring disparities evident within specific racial/ethnic immigrant communities in New York City or elsewhere in the country.

RATIONALE

The rationale for this study was established in part over a decade ago when the Federal Government's Healthy People 2000 (HP2000) program set a target IMR of 7.0 per 1000 live births (NCHS, 1999). The average U.S. IMR in 1997 of 7.1 was close enough to meeting the 2000 targets which allowed the Healthy People program not only to revise baseline data on IMR for all groups, but also to set a new, lower IMR target of 4.5 per 1000 (Centers for Disease Control and Prevention [CDC], 2003) for 2010. However, success at the national level is not always a reflection of experiences at the state and local levels.

By 1998, NYC achieved a city-wide IMR average of 6.4 which exceeded the HP2000 target of 7.0 and was certainly lower than the national average of 7.2 (March of Dimes, 2002). However, after closer examination of the 1998-IMR for NYC and of the more comprehensive 1996-1999 period, all of which showed racial differences in IMR, various local community-based organizations (CBOs) and providers began to raise questions about the disparities that emerged among various population groups, because they serviced these ethnic groups for many years and knew that problems of access to services existed particularly among their immigrant clients (Browne, Graham & Hylton, 1986; Graham, 1989; Goodbridge & Mason, 2001). Providers and CBOs not only raised questions but they also offered recommendations regarding promising and proven approaches to eliminate the disparities in their communities (Caribbean Women's Health Association [CWHA], 2000; Moses, 2000; Mason, 2001; Association of Perinatal Networks of New York [APNNY], 2002). Subsequently, New York City Department of Health (NYCDOH) released preliminary reports, indicating that despite a citywide IMR average of 6.9, there were population subgroups in the City for whom infant mortality rates were indeed much higher than the citywide average, along with draft action plans to reduce the disparities (NYCDOH, 2001). Later, with assistance from the Federal level (USDHHS, 2002), formal reports were then issued (Frieden, 2002) which became blueprints for action (NYCDOH, 2002) that targeted specific immigrant subgroups for intensive services to improve prenatal and neonatal health care services.

In a city of immigrants such as New York, media reports of high infant mortality rates among specific racial ethnic immigrant groups and the extent to which infants from these groups bore the burden of IMR disparities (Lipton, 2002; Johnson, 2000; Best, 2000) led to growing concern. Therefore, this study was undertaken in an effort to determine primarily what health disparities existed in the area of IMR in NYC and to explore possible approaches that could be taken towards eliminating those disparities. However, in addition to concerns about which groups were affected there was also a question regarding the specific neighborhoods, if any, in which the highest rates were found, and further, what were the contributing factor(s).

Therefore, the purpose of this study was twofold. First, the study used the NYCDOH reports to identify those groups in the City that had the highest IMR. Then, focused discussions were conducted with women from those groups in search of causal factors contributing to, or associated with, their higher IMR, with the goal of finding new explanations for this recent trend. Second, this study also compared IMRs between NYC and the countries of origin of those ethnic immigrant groups with the highest IMR concentrations in the City, to determine any particular trends, given the facility with which the many aspects of health (physical, social, economic, cultural and otherwise) move easily across and beyond borders, due to the facility of air travel and transnational identities and cultures (Bayne-Smith, 1996). Finally this paper concludes with specific recommendations of:

a. Identification, evaluation and use of successful models for strategic interventions to improve birth outcomes, and to eliminate disparities in IMR among various population groups in NYC, and
b. Recommendations for social work regarding service delivery to specific populations.

METHODOLOGY

Sample Selection

For Quantitative Data

Based on data compiled from NYCDOH, those ethnic groups with the highest IMRs in NYC were identified. This group represented a dozen countries:

10 in the circum-Caribbean region, and two from Africa. The sample on which quantitative data was drawn, consisted of only groups from the ten Caribbean countries with IMRs that were closest to or higher than the citywide average.

For Qualitative Data

It was decided to limit the qualitative sample of focus group participants to only Caribbean groups because of issues of access to, and facility of interaction with, Caribbean women. Therefore the qualitative focus group sample consisted only of mothers from those five Caribbean countries, identified as having the highest IMRs. The focus group sample was limited only to those women from the five countries with the highest IMRs (per 1000 births) because none of the remaining five countries had more than 500 births in 2000. Over-sampling of participants for the five groups being studied was done to establish focus groups of 8-10 women with common characteristics such as age, SES, country of origin, culture and language who could interact in a discussion around maternal child health issues.

Data Collection

Quantitative

Existing statistical data was collected on: the immigrant population of NYC, as well as the infant mortality rates for all boroughs of NYC from: New York City Department of City Planning (NYCDCP), NYCDOH, Census data, the Infoshare Database (*www.Infoshare.org*) and from local offices of the March of Dimes, Inc., to determine specific groups and neighborhoods in the City with the highest IMR concentrations. Additional data was obtained from NYCDOH that established IMR by race/ethnicity/immigrant group and selected maternal birthplaces (Li, 2000–NYCDOH, Special Statistical Analysis).

Qualitative

Factors identified as contributing to higher IMR among Caribbean immigrants were obtained by focus group research.

Data Analysis

Quantitative

Analysis of these various data sets was conducted to obtain frequency counts on the size of the immigrant population in NYC, and of IMR by maternal birthplace. The goal was to explore patterns of high IMR, across the various data sets to determine consistent concentrations of higher IMR among groups or neighborhoods, particularly minority and subspecial immigrant populations in the City. Investigations were also conducted to find patterns of increased risk factors for infant death among this population such as incidence of low birth weight, receipt of late or no prenatal care, percent of births by insurance coverage, race/ethnicity and neighborhood of residence.

Comparisons were then made of IMRs between NYC and countries of origin for the selected immigrant groups. Measurements of NYC-IMR risk factors are based on data from the NYC Department of Health. Country of origin IMR and related risk factors were taken from the World Health Organization 2001 Report on health conditions in the Americas (Alleyne, 2002).

Qualitative

Four separate groups were convened of 10 women each: one with women from Haiti, another with women from Jamaica, another from Guyana, and another from Puerto Rico. A fifth group of eight women from Trinidad and Tobago was convened. Each of the five focus groups was held with women from a different country because (a) the Caribbean is not a homogeneous, mono-cultural or mono-lingual region, and (b) the women represented immigrant groups with the highest IMRs (per 1000 live births) in NYC. The groups were assembled to achieve as much cohesiveness as possible on the basis of age (all teens, as opposed to those 20-39 years of age), ethnicity, and language. The only constant criteria common to all the groups: participants had to have had at least one pregnancy. In the interest of homogeneity which facilitates group discussion, the following focus groups were assembled: one Jamaican and one Puerto Rican group consisting of women ages 17-19, one group each of women from Haiti, Guyana and Trinidad/Tobago that consisted of women ages 20-32. All group sessions were conducted in English with the exception of the Haitian group, which was conducted in Creole.

Discussions focused on possible causative factors contributing to higher IMRs specifically in two areas: (a) Barriers/Issues of access to care both in NYC and at home and, (b) Cultural practices and health behaviors related to pregnancy. The recruitment and registration of women as potential participants in the discussion groups, included collection of basic demographic information including age, address, ethnic/racial group with which they most identified, level of education, availability of supports and resources. Using this information, participants were selected and invited to participate in a focus group with other women who shared similar characteristics of age, ethnic identification, education, and social networks. Great effort was made to assemble groups that achieved the highest level of compatibility among participants. Each focus group session was observed by a participant observer who was there to detect nonverbal reactions in addition to the audiotape, and an in-room note-taker. Both the in-room note-taker and the participant observer were fluent in the culture and language of the groups they participated in and took notes on. They then worked together to combine the observer's impressions, the recorder's notes and the transcribed tapes into one document. That document was then analyzed for frequency of comments and concerns of the focus group participants.

RESULTS

Quantitative

According to the NYCDCP, a third of NYC's population consists of foreign-born residents (New York City Department of City Planning [NYCDCP], 2000) (see Figure 1). This large immigrant population holds several critical implications for Social Work in particular and for the City in general in terms of immigrant access to culturally and linguistically appropriate health and other social and support services.

The process of immigration and settlement is one that is naturally shaped by kinship networks. As a result, new immigrants to the City move into immigrant enclaves where there is an existing concentration of people from their homelands. A summary report of vital statistics from NYCDOH for year 2000 provides information on IMR by borough and by specific neighborhoods (Figure 2, NYC–Residents, 2000). This figure indicates that the infant death rate for NYC as a whole was 6.7 per 1000, which is better than the HP2000 goal of 7 but above the HP2010 goal of 4.5. The concern here is that IMR are not uniform throughout the city. The IMR is clearly lower in Manhattan (5.0), Staten Island (6.1) and Queens (5.8), than the city average of 6.7. However, the overall NYC IMR of 6.7 in 2000 was surpassed for the Borough of Brooklyn (6.9) and for the Bronx (7.4). Further, the highest rates in Brooklyn are in the neighborhoods of: Bedford Stuyvesant-Crown Heights (10.8), East Flatbush-Flatbush (9.8), East New York (8.9), and Canarsie-Flatlands (8.7). In the Bronx the highest IMR rates are in the neighborhoods of Kingsbridge-Riverdale (10.8), Northeast Bronx (8.7), and Hunts Point-Mott Haven (8.4). According to NYC Department of City Planning, these neighborhoods in Brooklyn and the Bronx are immigrant enclave neighborhoods that experienced a consistent increased flow of new immigrants between 1983 and 1994 (NYCDCP, 1996).

FIGURE 1. Total Population by Nativity, New York City, 1990-2000–Native and Foreign Born

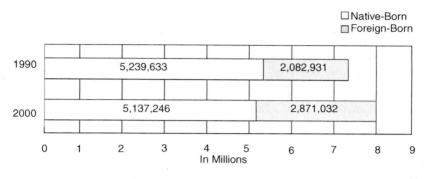

Distribution of Population by Nativity
1990-2000

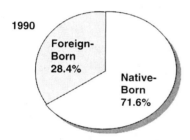

Total Population: 7,322,564

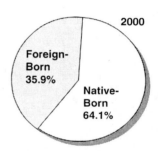

Total Population: 8,008,278

Source: New York City Department of City Planning

IMR by race in NYC follows the national pattern in which infant deaths are highest for Blacks, followed by Hispanics and lowest for Asians (Matthews, Menacker & MacDorman, 2002). However, very little attention is paid to the fact that, as a group, neither Blacks nor Hispanics are homogeneous. Local advocacy efforts by ethnic organizations to improve cultural and linguistic services in health care delivery have increased awareness, particularly for the mainstream, that among Blacks and Hispanics in NYC there are many different ethnic immigrant subgroups who speak a variety of languages (Graham, 2004). A

FIGURE 2. New York City Residents, 2000

Borough	UHF Neighborhood	Total Live Births	Number of Deaths	Infant Mortality	Neighborhood-borough/NYC
Manhattan		**19,813**	**99**	**5.0**	**0.75**
	Washington Heights-Inwood	4,272	22	5.1	0.77
	Central Harlem-Morningside Hts.	2,321	21	9.0	1.35
	East Harlem	1,771	17	9.6	1.44
	Upper West Side	2,652	5	1.9	0.28
	Upper East Side	2,737	12	4.4	0.66
	Chelsea-Clinton	1,123	7	6.2	0.93
	Gramercy Park-Murray Hill	1,159	2	1.7	0.26
	Greenwich Village-Soho	758	3	4.0	0.59
	Union Square-Lower East Side	2,575	6	2.3	0.35
	Lower Manhattan	361	4	11.1	1.66
Staten Island		**5,899**	**36**	**6.1**	**0.91**
	Port Richmond	984	6	6.1	0.91
	Stapleton-St. George	1,689	18	10.7	1.59
	Willowbrook	999	4	4.0	0.60
	South Beach-Tottenville	2,225	8	3.6	0.54
Bronx		**21,648**	**161**	**7.4**	**1.11**
	Kingsbridge-Riverdale	1,018	11	10.8	1.62
	Northeast Bronx	2,060	18	8.7	1.31
	Fordham-Bronx Park	4,495	37	8.2	1.23
	Pelham-Throgs Neck	3,880	17	4.4	0.66
	Crotona-Tremont	4,097	29	7.1	1.06
	High Bridge-Morrisania	3,836	30	7.8	1.17
	Hunts Point-Mott Haven	2,255	19	8.4	1.26
Brooklyn		**39,523**	**274**	**6.9**	**1.04**
	Greenpoint	2,332	13	5.6	0.83
	Williamsburg-Bushwick	3,732	23	6.2	0.92
	Downtown-Heights-Slope	2,726	20	7.3	1.10
	Bedford Stuyvesant-Crown Heights	5,353	58	10.8	1.62
	East New York	3,020	27	8.9	1.34
	Sunset Park	2,409	6	2.5	0.37
	Borough Park	6,112	19	3.1	0.47
	East Flatbush-Flatbush	5,389	53	9.8	1.47
	Canarsie-Flatlands	2,532	22	8.7	1.30
	Bensonhurst-Bayridge	2,442	13	5.3	0.80
	Coney Island-Sheepshead Bay	3,472	20	5.8	0.86
Queens		**28,517**	**164**	**5.8**	**0.86**
	Long Island City-Astoria	2,814	17	6.0	0.90
	West Queens	7,632	42	5.5	0.82
	Flushing-Clearview	2,623	15	5.7	0.86
	Bayside-Littleneck	522	3	5.7	0.86
	Ridgewood-Forest Hills	2,969	5	1.7	0.25
	Fresh Meadows	1,180	5	4.5	0.67
	Southwest Queens	3,772	11	2.9	0.44
	Jamaica	3,763	35	9.3	1.39
	Southeast Queens	1,917	18	9.4	1.41
	Rockaway	1,302	13	10.0	1.49
New York City*		**125,563**	**839**	**6.7**	

Source: New York City Department of Health Office of Vital Statistics. *Total live births and infant deaths for New York City included non-New York City residents.

March 2000 release from the Office of Vital Statistics of NYCDOH provided infant mortality data disaggregated by selected maternal places of birth (See Figure 3). That breakdown indicated that all IMRs closest to, or higher than, the citywide average occurred largely among infants born to mothers from countries that were predominantly in the circum-Caribbean region. Figure 3 indicates that the highest IMR by mother's birthplace were found in Haiti (13.9), Jamaica (9.4), "Other" Caribbean Countries (8.3), and Puerto Rico (8.0), all of which surpassed the NYC IMR of 6.7. It is important to note that the "Other" category includes only the Caribbean region countries of: Panama, Grenada, Barbados, St. Lucia and St. Vincent. However, NYCDOH explains that they were collapsed into one as each of those countries had fewer than 500 births in 2000.

Given the high levels of IMR among specific groups in the City, a primary concern is, how do we gain a better understanding of the problem? An initial step was to compare IMR for the identified groups both here as well as in their countries of origin. NYC IMR data for the selected groups was compared to international reports on IMR taken from the World Health Organization's 2001 Report on Health Conditions in the Americas (Alleyne, 2002). Using these two data sources, a comparison was made between the IMR of those groups identified as having the highest IMR in NYC and the IMR in their country of origin. Figure 4 provides a comparison indicating that IMR for Haitians in NYC in 2000 was (13.9), but (80.3) in Haiti in 2000; the IMR for Jamaicans in NYC was (9.4) in 2000 but (24.5) in Jamaica that same year; and the IMR for Panamanians in NYC was (11.0) in 1996-1998 and (16.8) in Panama in 1998.

Qualitative

The next step taken towards gaining a better understanding of the IMR problem among select immigrant groups from the Caribbean was to conduct focus groups. One important fact that resulted from the recruitment and registration of focus group participants, is that 65% of focus group participants had 12 years or less of education. This finding was consistent with similar information from NYCDOH which also indicated that among immigrant women with higher IMRs, 55% of them qualified for public insurance (Medicaid) in NYC to pay for their prenatal care (Li, 2003 NYCDOH-Special Statistical Analysis).

Throughout the group sessions two overarching themes repeatedly surfaced. The first revolved around difficulties experienced with health care systems and institutions and the lack of access to health care, both at home and in the U.S. The second theme was an acknowledgement of the impact of cultur-

FIGURE 3. Infant Mortality by Selected Maternal Place of Birth, 2000. Live Births, Infants Deaths and Infant Mortality Rate (IMR) by Mother's Birthplace, New York City, 2000 (Ordered by Highest IMR)

Birthplace	Live Births	Infant Deaths	IMR
Haiti	2,292	32	13.9
Jamaica	3,856	36	9.4
Other*	1,810	15	8.3
Puerto Rico	11,775	93	8.0
United Kingdom	638	5	7.8
Ghana	588	4	6.8
Nigeria	612	4	6.5
Trinidad & Tobago	1,913	12	6.3
Pakistan	1,419	9	6.3
Peru	517	3	5.8
Guyana	2,627	15	5.7
NYC Total	125,563	839	6.7

FIGURE 4. IMR by Ethnic Group in NYC and Country of Origin. IMR by Selected Groups–NYC, 1996-2000 and Country of Origin 1997-2000

Group	IMR-NYC	IMR-Country of Origin
Haiti	13.9 (2000)	80.3 (2000)
Jamaica	9.4 (2000)	24.5 (2000)
Puerto Rico	8.0 (2000)	10.6 (1999)
Trinidad & Tobago	6.3 (2000)	17.1 (1997)
Guyana	5.7 (2000)	22.2 (1998)
Panama	11.0 (1996-1998)	16.8 (1998)
Grenada	9.5 (1996-1998)	not available
Barbados	9.9 (1996-1998)	12.8 (1999)
St. Lucia	13.2 (1996-1998)	15.0 (1999)
St. Vincent	9.8 (1996-1998)	15.7 (2000)

ally influenced beliefs and health behaviors on utilization of the traditional western biomedical model. Figures 5 and 6 provide a summary of the most frequent responses from focus group participants. It is important to note in Figure 5, that one of the NYC barriers is difficulty with English for many immigrants. While it was expected that this would be a major concern for the Haitian group it also surfaced as a concern for 40% of the Puerto Rican group and 25% of the Jamaican group as well. That language presents a significant problem among English-speaking groups such as Jamaicans may very well be a function of educational levels which, based on data collected during recruitment of focus group participants, indicated that two-thirds of recruits had 12 years or less of schooling. In Figure 6, it is necessary to take note of the belief that while pregnancy has a physical component it does not require early prenatal care as long there was no pain. This belief was held primarily by the younger focus groups (Jamaican and Puerto Rican), rather than the other groups of older women from Haiti, Guyana and Trinidad/Tobago.

CULTURAL BELIEFS AND PRACTICES ABOUT PREGNANCY

Figure 5 captures the socioeconomic profile of the Caribbean population in NYC. This is a vibrant, productive and ambitious group that includes many middle class owners of businesses, professionals and the upwardly mobile. In addition, they also consist of a large proportion that are unskilled, and who are unable to speak English well. While they tend to find employment within the economy of their ethnic enclaves, these small ethnic community businesses are unable to offer them and their families employment-based health insurance. As a result they are unable to access health care services and are subject to the social ills and adverse health outcomes that beset the poor. Consequently, many women in the focus groups commented that: "Whether here or at home, going to the doctor requires some form of payment which I do not have, therefore I will use some of those remedies which I grew up with and which cost very little." Several women also captured the difficulty of communicating with providers: "I sometimes do not really understand what they are telling me at the clinic and they don't seem to understand me so unless I really have a problem, I prefer not to go."

Figure 6 focuses on culturally influenced beliefs and health behaviors. Focus group participants represented the health beliefs and practices of Caribbean people which are a mixture of traditional folk health and mainstream medical practices. While middle class Caribbean immigrants, in part because of greater financial accessibility, utilize mainstream western medical systems more readily, they are not the majority of immigrants. The post-1980 Caribbean migration came from working and lower class backgrounds; they are a hard working, spiritual people and they are more likely to rely on cheaper, more readily available folk medicine as well as on family supports during times of illness (Graham, 1989). It was therefore not surprising to hear comments from focus group participants such as: "It is so hard to be far from family during the time you are pregnant as you need the support of somebody who is like your mother to help you at that time." "I was lucky to get into a program for pregnant women run by the Caribbean Women's and I did have a woman come to my house after the baby was born and she was like a mother to me,

FIGURE 5. Access to Care Issues in Country of Origin and in NYC

Country of Origin	NYC
Rural areas = scarcity of health providers	Immigration reform and fear of deportation
Lack of fees to pay doctors	Lack of health insurance and Medicaid ineligibility
Transportation	Language barriers
Insufficient # of clinics to serve the poor in urban areas	Cultural insensitivity of large health care systems
Ready availability of home remedies	Cost of prescription meds
	Lack of social supports

Source: Focus Group Research Results-CWHA

FIGURE 6. Culturally Influenced Beliefs and Health Behaviors Related to Pregnancy

Beliefs	Health Behaviors
• **I am pregnant not sick, I do not need a doctor. Pregnancy has:**	• **I am pregnant, a state of being that is handled within the context of family. The pregnant woman seeks:**
– A physical component and if there is no pain all is well	– Spiritual guidance to meet challenges of raising a child
– A spiritual component which requires that mother maintain a positive spirit to infuse child with a spirit of joy	– Education from elders to learn proper child care
– A dietary component which requires the woman to eat certain foods for its perceived effect on the character, development and personal attributes of the child	

Source: Focus Group Research Results-CWHA

showing me a lot of things, and she prayed with me, but it was a special program and it did not last very long."

DISCUSSION

In view of the above findings it was also important to look at what the literature said about causes of infant mortality both in the U.S. and in the Caribbean. On the one hand, the National Center for Health Statistics (NCHS), a U.S. agency, has identified five leading causes of infant mortality: congenital anomalies, short gestation, sudden infant death syndrome (SIDS), respiratory distress syndrome (RDS) and maternal complications, all essentially concerned with poor birth outcomes (NCHS, 1998). Over the course of the last decade, several other studies have offered modifications of the conventional NCHS classification system, and these more recent explanations include the role of other causes particularly pre-maturity and birth-process related infant mortality as well as obstetric conditions and perinatal infections (Dolfus, Patteta, Siegel & Cross, 1990; Sowards, 1999). On the other hand, research on causative factors contributing to the high levels of IMR in various countries in the Caribbean and Latin American provides a long and varied list that ranges from issues such as economic performance and external debt to birth spacing and the nutritional status of pregnant women (Brittain, 1992; Blau, 1986; Hojman, 1994).

A striking aspect of all the explanations offered, whether they are U.S. or Caribbean focused, whether they place blame on poor birth outcomes or poor conditions in the country being discussed, is the underlying connecting thread of poverty and low educational levels among those groups with highest IMR both in NYC, across the U.S. and in the Caribbean (Henderson, 2000; Christiansen, 1996; Latin American Weekly Report Newsletter [LAWRN], Dec. 1995; LAWRN, Aug. 1995). This connection between infant mortality, poverty and low levels of education is also born out by our discussion groups. For example, in response to probing about the early and frequent use of private doctors in their countries of origin, every group dismissed that as a practice available only to the "better off" urban woman. For the most part participants reported that they, their family and friends waited on the limited availability of openings for new patients in the clinics located "in town" in order to receive any health services including prenatal care if it were necessary.

It is not uncommon for many of the privileged members of Caribbean society to fly to North America or Europe for high technology health care services or pay for the highest level of pregnancy-related care in their countries of origin (Aarons, 1999). Not so for those who are poor. Their situation is the same there as it is in NYC which is the new home for large numbers of poor people from the Caribbean who came to the U.S. in search for more opportunities than they had at home. When the more privileged migrate from the Caribbean they are more likely within a few years of acculturation and familiarization with the new terrain to move into middle management positions which will provide the kind of health benefits that facilitate access to private providers in NYC and other parts of the U.S.

CONCLUSION

Increasingly, national policy efforts have been aimed at providing targeted services to specific populations (HRSA, 2003). This kind of effort at the national level as well as the preceding results and discussion suggest that if we are to eliminate infant mortality disparities among the identified immigrant groups in NYC and elsewhere in the country, a major national effort is now needed. There has to be a national effort to seek out and conduct comprehensive evaluations of models that work (HRSA-BPHC, 1996; Delgado, 2002), with poor, underserved and immigrant communities. This will provide the evidence base for implementing more effective strategies that will serve to improve birth outcomes, reduce and eventually eliminate IMRs and other forms of health disparities at the local level.

Over and above health policy and programmatic efforts is the fact that at the root of health disparities, especially the excessive infant mortality rates among Caribbean groups in NYC, is their poverty levels. Consequently, the larger goal at both national and local levels must also be efforts to decrease and eventually eradicate the poverty that most assuredly predicts their impaired health.

Social Work agencies, in particular, especially those agencies that serve specific immigrant communities, must become instrumental in helping to establish community-based programs built on proven approaches such as the Health Keepers Model (Graham, to be published, 2004), that utilizes community health workers as a pool of staff drawn from the communities being served. This staffing pool must be trained to facilitate access to care for the poor. However, over and above the training that agencies provide, community health workers bring a moral authority that professionals lack, which they can use to encourage, motivate and insist that their countrywomen seek out and utilize health care services in a timely fashion that will serve to reduce the current levels of IMR among their group. Another concrete area for social work contribution must be in the development of English proficiency/health education programs as an initial step towards increasing access to, and use of, information, education and ultimately the health care services that will help to eliminate health disparities. Combined programs of English language proficiency and health education are of vital importance in that they will serve the dual purpose of increasing language skills that are critical to accessing services as well as to moving out of poverty.

The use of community health workers is highly recommended because of the beliefs and behaviors expressed by focus group participants. As summarized in Figure 6, women repeatedly commented on the spiritual component of pregnancy, the need for education from older women about childcare and the need for spiritual guidance to properly raise their children. This points to critical ingredients and changes required in social work and health care programming as we move to eliminate health disparities in infant mortality, and that has to do with the goal of meeting people where they are–physically, economically, culturally, socially and spiritually.

The comments from focus group participants (Figure 6) suggest that most promising approaches for improving IMR among the groups studied are those that are community-driven with peers and/or community women providing support to fellow residents of a community, to offer guidance and direction. These approaches must also be community-wide in scope and comprehensive in nature, as a woman trying to find somewhere to live, who has no information or referrals to accomplish that type of priority goal, will not keep prenatal care appointments. Social work programs and policies must now very boldly go so far as to ensure that immigrants become culturally competent to function in a large metropolitan area such as NYC, which is a radically different environment from the one they came from, if we are to increase the chances of healthy long lives for their children. If we listen to the women's concerns and we are serious about addressing this problem, then we will work to connect immigrants to a network of programs and services that will help them to acquire more education, better jobs and teach them how to create wealth, thereby elevating their socioeconomic status and the quality of life for them and for all of us.

The more formidable barriers for immigrant groups, as we move to eliminate disparities in infant mortality and other health areas that were identified by focus group participants summarized in Figure 5, have to do with policy reforms in the areas of immigration, welfare and health insurance/health care for all. Social Workers and others involved in the policy arena must be prepared for whatever windows of opportunity present themselves to push forward policies that will help to eliminate health disparities or, at the very least, reduce the burden for poor immigrant groups of color in the U.S. Policy level work must not lose sight of the fact that infant mortality among immigrant populations is the outcome of a number of causal factors stemming from the country of origin as well as factors that are U.S.- and NY-related (see Figure 5). Therefore, funding, both public and private, for elimination of IMR disparities has to address those various barriers and not focus solely on the provision of prenatal care.

This study is an initial start towards better understanding of high infant mortality incidence among immigrant groups of color living in NYC, and other large urban areas across the U.S. As such, it had limitations in that it relied on international data from external sources. The authors recommend that as we increase our efforts to eliminate high IMR and other health problems for the latest newcomers, there is a need for further research. We must conduct program assessment of various models of current maternal child health services being provided to immigrant groups in NYC and across the country. Analysis of the impact of promising approaches and effective results will enable us to find models that work in order to recommend strategic interventions towards the goal of improving infant mortality and birth outcomes for a variety of racial ethnic groups.

REFERENCES

Aarons, D.E. *Medicine and its alternatives: Caribbean medical care priorities.* The Hastings Center Report. July 1999; 29(4):23-27.

Alleyne, George. *Health situation in the Americas: Basic indicators–2001.* Geneva: World Health Organization. 2002.

Association of Perinatal Networks of New York in collaboration with the New York State Department of Health. Charting a course for perinatal health in New York State. *Bureau of Women's Health.* Nov. 7, 2001.

Bayne-Smith, Marcia A. *Race, gender and health.* California: Sage Publications, 1996.

Bayne-Smith, Marcia A. Ethnic organizations and the politics of multiculturalism: The case of Caribbean Americans. In John Stanfield, Ed. *Research in social policy,* Volume 4. pp. 145-171. JAI Press, Inc. 1996.

Best, T. Caribbean child survival in New York City: Unhealthy picture, infant mortality rate one of the highest. *The New York Carib News.* April 25, 2000.

Blau, D.M. Fertility, child nutrition and child mortality in Nicaragua. *Journal of Developing Areas.* 1986; 20:185-201.

Browne, R., Graham Y.J., Hylton D. Eds. *Delivering culturally compatible prenatal care services to immigrants: The Caribbean population in New York City.* Caribbean Women's Health Association, Inc. 1986.

Caribbean Women's Health Association Annual Report. (See also: Caribbean Women's Health Association's Campaign to Fight Infant Mortality, CWHA, Brooklyn, NY, August, 2000).

Casper, M.L., Barnett, E., Halverson, J.A., Elmes, G.A., Braham, V.E., Majeed, Z.A., Bloom, A.S., Stanley, S. *Women and heart disease: An atlas of racial and ethnic disparities in mortality,* Second Edition. Office for Social Environment and Health Research, West Virginia University, Morgantown WV: December, 2000.

Centers for Disease Control and Prevention, (CDC) HP2010 Database, National Vital Statistics System, Mortality and Natality. Feb. 2003. Objective 16-01C–Infant deaths.

Centers for Disease Control and Prevention National Vital Stats Reports Vol. 52, No. 3, Table 31, Page 92. Sept. 18, 2003.

Christiansen, S., Rosen, A. *Black infant mortality.* Briefing paper developed for Memorial Health System of South Bend, Indiana. The Family Connection of St. Joseph County, Inc. 1996.

Collins, J.W. Jr., Butler, A.G. Racial differences in prevalence of small-for-dates infants among college educated women. *Epidemiology* May, 1997. 8(3):315-7.

Delgado, Debra. *The PLAIN TALK Implementation Guide,* The Annie E. Casey Foundation 2002.

Dollfus. C., Patteta. M., Siegel. E., Cross. A.W. Infant mortality: A practical approach to the analysis of the leading causes of death and risk factors. *Pediatrics.* 1990; 86:176-183.

Frieden, Thomas R. *Infant mortality in NYC: Trends and strategies.* Department of Health and Mental Health, Mental Retardation and Alcoholism Services. May 16, 2002.

Goodbridge, A., Mason, M.A. Infant mortality in the Caribbean-American community. *Wadabagei: A Journal of the Caribbean and its Diaspora.* The Caribbean Research Center of Medgar Evers College, CUNY, Brooklyn, NY. 2001; 4:81-105.

Graham, Y.J. Maternal child health profile of the Caribbean American population in New York City: Establishing new lives. In Velta J. Clarke and E. Riviere, Eds. *Selected readings on Caribbean Americans in NYC.* Caribbean Research Center of Medgar Evers College, City University of New York. 1989.

Graham, Y.J., The Health Keepers Model. In Marcia Bayne-Smith, Yvonne Graham and Sally Guttmacher (Eds.). *Community based health organizations.* California: Jossey Bass, To be published in 2004.

Guyer, B., Freedman M.A, Strobino, D.M., Sondik, E.J. Annual summary of vital statistics: Trends in the health of Americans during the 20th Century. *Pediatrics,* Dec. 2000, Vol. 106:1307-1317.

Henderson, C.W. Study shows racial differences in mortality rates. Medical letter on the CDC and FDA, 02/07/2000.

Health Resources and Services Administration (HRSA), *RFA for targeted peer support model development and evaluation for caribbeans living with HIV?* AIDS, April, 2003.

Health Resources and Services Administration (HRSA)–Bureau of Primary Health Care (BPHC). *Models that work: A compendium of innovative primary health care programs for underserved and vulnerable populations.* 1996.

Hojman, D.E. *Economic and other determinants of infant and child mortality in small developing countries: The case of Central America and the Caribbean.* University of Liverpool, Institute of Latin American Studies. 1994; Research Paper 16.

Johnson, Wista Jean. Body politics. *The Village Voice.* September 20-26, 2000.

Kaufman & Joseph Fox. Health status of American Indian and Alaska native women. In Marcia Bayne-Smith (Ed.) *Race, gender and health,* California: Sage, 1996.

Klein, R.J., Hawk, S.A. *Statistical notes: Health status indicators: Definitions and national data.* Hyattsville, MD. Public Health Service; 1992:1.

Latin American Weekly Report Newsletter. *Ignore the high population growth scenario in Latin America at your peril.* Aug., 1995.

Latin American Weekly Report Newsletter. *Trends: Life expectancy, infant mortality improve: But UNICEF index points to effects of wide income disparities.* Dec., 1995.

Le, L.T., Kiely, J.L., Schoendorf, K.C. Birth-weight outcomes among Asian American and Pacific Islander subgroups in the U.S. *Int. J Epidemiol* Oct., 1996; 25 (5):973-9.

Li, Wenhui. New York City Department of Health. Selected characteristics of mothers by age, group and by selected Caribbean and African countries. 2000.

Lipton, E. More money sought to fight jumps in infant death rates. *New York Times.* Feb. 5, 2001.

March of Dimes. *Perinatal Profiles: Statistics for monitoring state maternal and infant health*–New York, 2002 Edition.

Mason, M.A. *Caribbean Women's Health Association. 2001 Report card on the health status of the Caribbean-American community in New York City: Time to eliminate the disparities.* An unpublished report produced by Caribbean Women's Health Association, May, 2000. (See also: Mason M.A. Infant Mortality in New York City's Caribbean-American community: CWHA's strategic intervention Initiatives to reduce the disparities. Caribbean Women's Health Association, Inc. Brooklyn. July 2002.)

Mathews, T.J., Menacker, F., MacDorman, M.F. Infant Mortality statistics from the 2000 period linked birth/infant death data set. *CDC-NVSR* 2002; 50(12):27pp.

McCloskey, Lois, et al. A community-wide infant mortality review: Findings and implications. *Public Health Reports*, 1999. Vol. 114.

McBarnette, L. Health status of African American women. In Marcia Bayne-Smith (Ed.) Race, gender and health, California: Sage, 1996.

MMWR. 1999, 48:849-857, Healthier Mothers and Babies–1900–1999. *JAMA*, 1999. Vol. 282.

MMWR. *Healthier mothers and babies.* 1999; 48:849-857.

MMWR. *Consensus set of health status indicators for the general assessment of community health status–United States.* MMWR. 1991;40:449-451.

Moses, NA. Dialogue on rising infant deaths in Brooklyn. *Caribbean Life.* April 18, 2000.

National Center for Health Statistics. The nation's health is up, but still lagging for poor, less educated. *Nation's Health* Sept., 1998; 29(8):36.

National Center for Health Statistics. Advance report of final mortality statistics, 1991. *Monthly Vital Stats Report.* 1993; 42(2) (suppl.).

NYC Department of City Planning. *The Newest New Yorkers,* 1996.

New York City Department of Health. Proposal for Infant Mortality Reduction. Phase III report blueprint for action. Draft, Community-Working document. Jn 8, 2001.

New York City Department of Health. Infant Mortality Reduction Initiative–Summary of Phase III Report–Blueprint for Action. May 31, 2002.

New York City Department of City Planning, 2000.

Rodgers, A., Vaughan, P. et al. The World Health Report–2002: Reducing Risks, Promoting healthy life. Geneva: World Health Organization, 2002.

Singh G.K., Yu S.M., Infant Mortality in he United States: Trends, differentials, and projections 1950 through 2010. *Am J Public Health.* 1995; 85(7): 957-964.

Sowards, K.A. What is the leading cause of infant mortality? A note on the interpretation of official statistics. *American Journal of Public Health,* 1999; 89: 1752-54.

U.S. Department of Health and Human Service Press Office. *Preventing infant mortality.* March 18, 2002.

U.S.DHHS. National Center for Health Statistics. HP2000 Progress Review-Maternal and infant health. May, 1999.

United Nations Development Programme. Human Development Report–2001. New York: UNICEF.

USDHHS, Heckler Report. (1985) Report of the secretary's task force on black and minority health. Washington, DC: Government Printing Office.

Vohr, B.R., Dusick, A., Steichen, J., Wright, L.L., Verter, J., Mele L. Neuro-developmental and functional outcome of extremely low birth weight (ELBW) infants. Pediatr Res 1998; 43:238A.

Confronting the Reality:
An Overview of the Impact of HIV/AIDS
on the Caribbean Community

Mary Spooner
Carol Ann Daniel
Annette M. Mahoney

SUMMARY. The most recent UNAIDS report (December 2003) estimates that approximately 5 million persons became infected with the HIV virus globally in 2003 alone, while 3 million persons died as a result of HIV/AIDS. What do these staggering numbers mean for the Caribbean population? Is the impact of HIV/AIDS the same among Caribbean immigrants in the United States as among the Caribbean population in the countries of origin? If so, what are the factors that promote the spread of HIV/AIDS among this population regardless of their geographic location? Finally, what can be done to reverse the growing infection rate that has made the Caribbean the second largest population to suffer from HIV/AIDS globally? In this paper the au-

Mary Spooner, PhD, is Program Evaluation Director, Holy Cross Children's Services, Clinton, MI.

Carol Ann Daniel, CSW, ABD, is Assistant Professor of Sociology at Brooklyn College, City University of New York.

Annette M. Mahoney, DSW, MS, is Assistant Professor at the Hunter College School of Social Work, City University of New York.

[Haworth co-indexing entry note]: "Confronting the Reality: An Overview of the Impact of HIV/AIDS on the Caribbean Community." Spooner, Mary, Carol Ann Daniel, and Annette M. Mahoney. Co-published simultaneously in *Journal of Immigrant & Refugee Services* (The Haworth Social Work Practice Press, an imprint of The Haworth Press, Inc.) Vol. 2, No. 3/4, 2004, pp. 49-67; and: *The Health and Well-Being of Caribbean Immigrants in the United States* (ed: Annette M. Mahoney) The Haworth Social Work Practice Press, an imprint of The Haworth Press, Inc., 2004, pp. 49-67. Single or multiple copies of this article are available for a fee from The Haworth Document Delivery Service [1-800-HAWORTH, 9:00 a.m. - 5:00 p.m. (EST). E-mail address: docdelivery@haworthpress.com].

http://www.haworthpress.com/web/JIRS
Digital Object Identifier: 10.1300/J191v2n03_04

thors explore sociocultural, attitudinal and gender-specific factors that place the Caribbean population at risk of the ongoing spread of HIV/AIDS. The authors make recommendations for a community involvement response to the HIV/AIDS epidemic that targets the individual, family and community to address the problem of HIV/AIDS in the Caribbean population. A community involvement model with its potential to reduce the negative impact of socio-structural factors, and attitudes towards victims of HIV/AIDS is recommended as a meaningful response to HIV/AIDS among the Caribbean population. *[Article copies available for a fee from The Haworth Document Delivery Service: 1-800-HAWORTH. E-mail address: <docdelivery@haworthpress.com> Website: <http://www.HaworthPress.com> © 2004 by The Haworth Press, Inc. All rights reserved.]*

KEYWORDS. HIV/AIDS, Caribbean, Caribbean immigrants

If we continue as we are, each year losing a little ground, this is where we will stand–a place of pain and sorrow, of unimaginable loss and of collective shame. Then together we will have failed to protect the vulnerable, voiceless, powerless, sick and orphaned. (Dr. Peter Piot, Executive Director, UNAIDS, October 2001, Melbourne, Australia)

No other disease has claimed the lives of victims in the 20th Century at as fast a rate as HIV/AIDS. The Black Death or bubonic plague–once considered to be the world's worst pandemic–will soon rank in second place to HIV/AIDS as the cause of death of the world's population. Globally, misconceptions about HIV/AIDS, its transmission and deadly impact on the world population have led to an increase in the prevalence of the disease with the potential to inflict numerous deaths worldwide.

The Caribbean region–defined as the chain of islands stretching from the Bahamas in the North to Trinidad and Tobago in the south and including Guyana on the South American mainland–is now considered to have the second highest rate of HIV prevalence in the world; Sub-Saharan Africa has the highest rate of prevalence. Since the first reported cases of AIDS in the Caribbean region in 1982, the disease has spread rapidly throughout the region (TransAfrica Forum, 2002).

Since the late 1970s when HIV/AIDS became recognized as an epidemic, 21.8 million persons have died worldwide (Bryan, February 6, 2002, North-South Center Update). The most recent report by the Joint United Nations Program on HIV/AIDS (UNAIDS, December 2003) estimates that there are 40 million HIV positive persons worldwide. The spread and impact of the disease has been dramatic. In 2003 alone, more than 5 million persons around the globe became infected with the virus and 3 million persons died as a result of HIV/AIDS or related complications of the illness (UNAIDS, 2003).

HIV infection continues to be prominent among men who have sex with men in the United States. Forty-six percent of men infected in 2001 were categorized by the Department of Health and Human Services as "men who have sex with men," while 27% of infections were due to "other/risk not identified" category, 13% due to intravenous drug use, 7% due to contact between heterosexuals and 6% due to "men who have sex with men and inject drugs." Among women, heterosexual contact remains the primary means of HIV infection and black women continue to be the largest group of women infected by the virus (Department of Health and Human Services, 2001). Decline in the prevalence of HIV infection in the United States since 1996 is not reflected in the population of women as the disease continues to rise among women (Department of Health and Human Services, 2000, 2001).

Despite projections that by the year 2010 there will be 45 million newly infected victims, there is still hope that 29 million new HIV infections might be prevented through implementation of strategic policies to stop the progress of HIV/AIDS. The quality of life has been better for victims in developed countries like the United States than in developing countries. Some African countries have experienced an AIDS related death rate of up to 25% of their population (Bryan, 2002). The disparity in the progress in the fight against HIV/AIDS between developed and developing countries emphasizes the inequality in the response of governments to this debilitating disease. The lives of many victims of HIV/AIDS in the United States have been extended while many victims of the disease in countries such as Africa face death within a short time of contracting the disease. The present disparity in global consciousness and public response to this deadly disease raises many moral and ethical questions.

In the context of a world that is increasingly globalized, the response of the developed world to the plight of developing countries in Africa and the Caribbean cannot be differentiated. The key to success in fighting HIV/AIDS among the Caribbean population is to understand the patterns of behavior among this population. Regardless of where members of an ethnic group reside, it is important to focus on the value systems and traditions of the group in designing effective preventive programs (Gray, 1997). It therefore becomes imperative that the response to HIV/AIDS in the Caribbean community focuses on responding to the cultural lifestyles of the population wherever that population resides. It would be foolhardy to attempt to address this population's ills in the same manner as those of populations that do not exhibit the same cultural mores and patterns of behavior.

This paper looks at the prevalence of HIV/AIDS among the Caribbean population in the Caribbean and here in the United States. It argues for a response to the epidemic among this population as a group rather than one determined by geographic location. Consideration of the response to the Caribbean population as a culturally-specific group allows for development of more effective policies that increase the likelihood of arresting the spread of the disease within this population and extending the quality of life of those persons already infected. In considering an effective response to HIV/AIDS among the Caribbean population, theoretical approaches to behavior change are vital and their relevance must be understood in the context of the population to be served.

THEORETICAL APPROACHES TO HIV/AIDS INTERVENTION

High-risk sexual behavior has been identified as a key factor in the spread of HIV/AIDS. Since the HIV/AIDS crisis has deepened in the United States, social behaviorists have sought to employ various theories of behavior and behavior change to develop effective intervention models that would change high-risk behavior. In a literature that is continuously growing, three theories have positively impacted the behavioral research on HIV/AIDS–the Health Belief Model (Becker, 1974, 1988), the Theory of Reasoned Action (Ajzen & Fishbein, 1980), and Social Cognitive Learning Theory (Bandura, 1977).

Influenced by the theories of Lewin, the Health Belief Model seeks to predict an individual's health-related behavior in the context of patterns of belief. Hence, individual perceptions, modifying behaviors, and likelihood of action in combination cause action if accompanied by a rational alternative course of action. Developed in 1967, the Theory of Reasoned Action provides a framework to study attitudes toward patterns of behavior. It establishes that a person's action is determined by behavioral intent that represents a combination of attitude and subjective norm. Reasoned Action Theory is most effective when there is volitional control of one's behavior and there are no intervening environmental barriers. The premise of Social Cognitive Learning Theory is that behavior change is difficult when left to someone who has no clear intent or reason to adapt alternative patterns of behavior. According to Bandura (1977), "Learning would be exceedingly laborious, not to mention hazardous, if people had to rely solely on the effects of their own actions to inform them what to do. Fortunately, most human behavior is learned observationally through modeling: from observing others one forms an idea of how new behaviors are performed, and on later occasions this coded information serves as a guide for action" (p. 22). A key element of these three theories is the development of a better understanding of how change in human behavior might be achieved through attitudinal changes and subsequent modeling of desired behavior to influence required change.

Effective change in patterns of sexual behavior among the Caribbean population requires a model that effectively addresses environmental constraints. Among the Caribbean population where patterns of behavior are deeply embedded in learned behavior through oral tradition and shared images, the process of changing high-risk behavior among the Caribbean population is complex. Change is therefore best promoted if the environmental constraints are clearly identified and addressed. Environmental challenges for the Caribbean population include socio-structural and attitudinal issues as well as gender relations and, particularly in the United States, the problem of racism.

One model that shows promise for addressing environmental challenges is the community involvement model proposed by Ramirez-Valles (2002). Community involvement is defined by Ramirez-Valles (2002) as "a construct indicating individuals' unpaid work on behalf of others or a collective good and in the context of a formal or semi-formal organization and social networks, i.e., outside the home and the family" (p. 391). This model is significant in responding to HIV/AIDS populations because it encourages consistent use of condoms by male partners, the most effective means of preventing the spread of HIV aside from abstinence. Moreover, it encompasses the components that mitigate the negative impact of socio-structural and attitudinal factors and gender inequities. It also draws on the principles of the three theories mentioned previously to provide the tools used in community involvement to facilitate learning and behavior change.

In the process of doing community work, participants–persons who are HIV positive, their loved one and families–have the opportunity to share their experiences, learn safer sexual practices as well as providing emotional support for each other. These aspects of behavioral change might facilitate a transition in infected persons' behaviors but at the same time it contributes to the building of a community that is more understanding and less judgmental of those infected by the virus. "Through involvement in collective action, individuals increase their understanding of the agents that facilitate or inhibit the capacity to be proactive in their efforts to change their own health and the health of their community" (Zimmerman, 1995). In addition, individuals "produce their own knowledge and incorporate it into their own realities" (Ramirez-Valles, 2002, p. 394). The presence of strong familial and kinship networks among the Caribbean population provides a critical prerequisite that has the potential to enhance the effectiveness of the community involvement model. The model can be particularly advantageous in maintaining family and kinship bonds that are often weakened when persons are diagnosed as HIV positive but also in counteracting high-risk sexual behavior with more responsible behavior.

UNDERSTANDING HIV/AIDS IN THE CARIBBEAN

The spread of HIV/AIDS among the Caribbean population is promoted through continued engagement in high-risk sexual behavior, largely learned from observation of behavior patterns of the larger group or by compliance with what might be perceived as social and cultural expectations. Social norms that encourage early sexual engagement and promiscuity among some segments of the population, for example, could be considered a major contributor to HIV/AIDS transmission. Hence, it is important to understand the environmental context of Caribbean societies.

According to Caribbean Epidemiology Centre (CAREC), by the end of 2001, governments in the English-speaking Caribbean officially reported a total of 20,309 cases of AIDS. Lack of standardized reporting or failure to report cases of HIV/AIDS, however, makes it difficult to get a true picture of the real impact of the disease on the Caribbean population. Official reports place the actual number of people living with AIDS in the Caribbean between 360,000 (World Bank Group, 2003) and over 500,000 (UNAIDS, 2003).

Almost 50% of new HIV infections in the Caribbean are said to occur among persons aged 15 to 24 years. According to the World Bank Group (2003), "the affected age groups are the core of the labor force. Among men, the majority of AIDS cases are in the 30-34 and 25-29 year-old age group; among women, the majority of cases are in the 25-29 year-old age bracket, followed by the 30-34 age group" (p. 1).

The variety in the patterns of social and economic development among Caribbean countries affects the rate at which the HIV disease spreads between Caribbean countries and other regions (Nicholls et al., undated publication). Haiti presently has the highest rate of HIV/AIDS among adults followed by the Bahamas (see Fig. 1). In 2001, UNAIDS estimated that the prevalence rate among adults aged 15-49 years in Haiti was 6%. Approximately 4% of the adults in the Bahamas, aged 15-49 years, were infected with HIV/AIDS (PAHO/CAREC/UNAIDS, 2002).

The rate of infection in the Dominican Republic was reported to be in the region of 46% of sex workers and 2.5% of the Dominican population aged 15-49 years (see Fig 1). Approximately 85% of all the cases of HIV in the Caribbean are among Haitians and Dominicans (World Bank, 2003). Lower but still troubling, rates of infection persist in the English-speaking Caribbean is-

FIGURE 1. HIV Prevalence Rates in Adults 15-49 Years, 2001

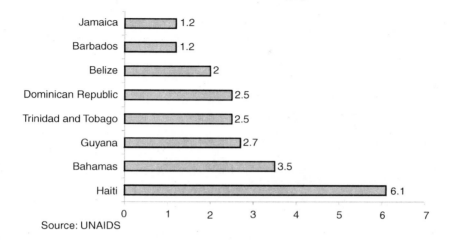

Source: UNAIDS

lands. For example, almost 40% of deaths among young males in St. Vincent and the Grenadines have been attributed to AIDS.

HIV/AIDS is transmitted primarily through sexual contact among heterosexual couples in the Caribbean. According to Jamaica AIDS Support (2002), "Contrary to popular myth limiting risk of infection to homosexuality and prostitution, for well over fifteen years heterosexual transmission has been the major reported factor in the Caribbean epidemic (64% of AIDS mortality) with combined reported homosexual and bisexual transmission representing a distinct minority (11%), and an unknown group at 17%" (p. 1).

Estimates of male-to-male sexual transmission of HIV/AIDS in the Caribbean region are likely to be conservative since male-to-male transmission remains largely underreported because of the stigma attached to homosexual behavior. Male-to-female ratio of AIDS remains at 2:1 with infection rates growing more quickly among females. CAREC reports that for the five years prior to 2000, "the absolute number of AIDS cases among women increased 1.7 times. There have been more male AIDS cases reported for all age groups, with the exception of the 15-19 group, which suggests that adolescent girls may be especially vulnerable" (p. 1).

HIV/AIDS is also prevalent in sectors such as the tourism industry, an industry on which the economies in the Caribbean are heavily reliant. While the industry provides lucrative income to those who work in the sector and a healthy balance of payments for the Caribbean economy, it also exposes many tourism workers to the likelihood of contracting HIV/AIDS. Sex tourism draws young people of both genders and several age groups into the trade on a part-time or full-time basis to supplement falling incomes. " 'Beach boys' or 'rent-a-dreads,' young men who are part of the sex trade, have become staples throughout the Caribbean" (Bryan, 2002 p. 3). Transmission of HIV/AIDS is therefore not uncommon among commercial sex workers such as beach boys, dancers and call girls working in the tourism sector. As Figueroa (2001) points out, "The high rates of HIV infection among those most at risk is a matter of concern because this provides a pool which contributes to HIV transmission in the general population . . . " (p. 19).

GENDER RELATIONS IN CARIBBEAN SOCIETIES

Significant inequities in gender relations among the Caribbean population relate to an imbalance in the distribution of power, economic and social resources. Many women and girls are often forced by necessity to undertake sex work to support their families often because of their lack of other sources of income. In circumstances where women are financially dependent on men it might be difficult for women to negotiate safer sexual practices and to protect themselves from the HIV virus.

Gender inequity also occurs as a result of the process of socialization of boys and girls. Among some segments of the population boys are allowed to engage in promiscuous behavior while girls are discouraged from sexual encounters before marriage. The result is that girls are less likely to develop the skills for negotiating safe sexual practices such as condom use.

Religious beliefs that prohibit the use of contraceptives as well as commonly held views that relate condom use to promiscuity often prevent women from encouraging their partners to use condoms during intercourse. A woman in a steady relationship who insists on use of a condom may be suspected of being unfaithful to her partner and risks being abandoned or becoming a victim of domestic violence. A woman in a less permanent relationship who insists on condom use may raise suspicions of being a carrier of the HIV disease.

Social pressure also forces some women into heterosexual relationships to establish and maintain social standing in Caribbean society. In a society where women who fail to marry or to be part of an ongoing heterosexual relationship are looked upon suspiciously and often as failures, women often take unnecessary risks by standing in as mistresses to already married men or men who have no intention to establish a monogamous relationship.

Risk of exposure to HIV/AIDS is often a function of migrant women's vulnerability in new and unfamiliar surroundings. For women bold enough to seek a better life in a foreign country, high-risk behavior might be their only means of negotiating legal hurdles related to immigration status, for example. Women might engage in casual relationships with men they perceive to be in a position to help them to gain legal status in a country and such relationships become major units of transaction in establishing residency in a foreign country. In such cases women are vulnerable to exposure to HIV/AIDS as they have little control over what happens to them sexually and the conditions under which these sexual encounters take place.

As the major caregivers within Caribbean communities, a diagnosis of HIV brings overwhelming emotional and social consequences for women. When a woman becomes infected with HIV/AIDS she is no longer able to care for her herself or her family and various social problems become imminent. At the personal level, many women of childbearing age face the knowledge that expectations about childbearing might change and this can be devastating for them. This means that adjustments have to be made both at the personal and family levels. In communities where women gain family and community support, the impact might be greatly mitigated but overall individual, family, community and public support structures are required to fill the void.

FEMINIZATION OF HIV/AIDS AND ITS IMPACT ON CARIBBEAN SOCIETIES

There is noticeable disparity in the spread of HIV/AIDS in the Caribbean along gender lines. The evidence shows that more Caribbean women are affected by HIV/AIDS than Caribbean men. Women of childbearing years in the Caribbean region are the fastest-growing group of persons to be infected with HIV/AIDS. According to a recent World Bank Report (World Bank, 2003), "currently, the Caribbean region has one of the highest rates of new AIDS cases among women in the Americas, reflecting the growing 'feminization' of the HIV/AIDS epidemic" (p. 1).

Except for Haiti and the Dominican Republic where men and women are equally impacted by HIV/AIDS, there is a clear disparity in the male/female ratio afflicted by the disease. According to a special report by *The Sun-Sentinel* (June 10, 2001), the ratio of female to male infection in Dominica is 3.6:1, in Barbados the ratio is 2.8:1, and in Trinidad, the ratio is 2.4:1. The rate of increase is particularly alarming among pregnant women. Haiti and Guyana experienced an infection rate among mothers of 7 to 8%.

Poverty plays a major role in the spread of HIV/AIDS in the Caribbean where women head an average of 35% of all Caribbean households with little, if any marketable skills for employment in the formal labor force. Additionally, in an economic structure where for decades assets such as land, were customarily passed to men, many women remain desperately poor. Among poor women, therefore, there is a high rate of dependence on men folk for financial support or to supplement their meager incomes. In some cases, women engage in serial relationships to optimize their economic earning potential. Women who are reliant on men for regular support are generally likely to acquiesce to their requests to engage in unprotected sex and hence raise their risk of exposure to HIV/AIDS. In many cases, unprotected sexual practices occur between young girls and older men who can provide the financial support required by poor disadvantaged adolescent girls.

HIV/AIDS has taken a deadly toll on the young and powerless in the Caribbean region. The youngest victims of HIV/AIDS in the Caribbean are the infants born to infected mothers. Some 25 to 30% of infected mothers were said to infect their children *in utero*, during their delivery or in the process of breast-feeding. More than 80,000 children have been orphaned as a result of AIDS in the Caribbean (Marquez, 2002). Equally alarming is the high prevalence of HIV infection among child prostitutes. For example, the United Nations Children Fund (UNICEF) reported that there are 50,000 infected child prostitutes in the Dominican Republic. In 2001, the Jamaican Ministry of Health reported 200 HIV positive and homeless children registered (*Sun-Sentinel*, June 10, 2001). By the end of 2002, UNAIDS estimated that there were 20,000 children under the age of 15 years living with HIV/AIDS in the Caribbean, 7,000 were newly infected and 7,000 died as a result (*Sun-Sentinel*, June 10, 2001).

HIV/AIDS IN THE CARIBBEAN DIASPORA–
THE CASE OF THE CITY OF NEW YORK

Patterns of behavior among the Caribbean population change very little upon migration. As a result HIV/AIDS rages not only in the countries of origin in the Caribbean, but also among the population of the Caribbean Diaspora. Hence, in cities like New York, the rate of HIV/AIDS infection remains alarming. In March 2000, the Office of AIDS Surveillance, New York City Department of Health reported HIV/AIDS rates of 46% among persons of Caribbean descent, compared to 27% among those of Latin American descent, 17% among those of East European/Soviet descent, 5% among those of Far/Near East descent, 3% among Africans and 2% among persons from other parts of the world (Office of AIDS Surveillance, New York City Department of Health, March 2000).

The magnitude of the HIV/AIDS problem within the Caribbean population is particularly noticeable in poorer areas of New York City. Crown Heights, which has been home to a significant population of Caribbean immigrants since the 1960s, has the highest number of cumulative diagnosed HIV/AIDS cases in the borough of Brooklyn, New York. Although only 12% of Brooklyn's population, Crown Heights accounts for 23% of the diagnosed AIDS cases in Brooklyn's adult/adolescent population. According to the Centers for Disease Control and Prevention (2000), Crown Heights has more people living with AIDS than the state of Indiana (AIDS & HIV Surveillance Report, CDC, 2000).

The high rate of HIV/AIDS cases in Crown Heights persists together with a high poverty rate. At 25%, the poverty rate of Crown Heights is higher than that of the entire borough of Brooklyn (20%) and doubles that of New York City (11%) (City of New York Office of Management and Budget, Department of City Planning, Fiscal Year 2001). However, income support is only 20.3% compared to Brooklyn's average of 25.5% and 21.8% for New York City, areas with greater populations than that of Crown Heights. This underutilization of services reflects the challenges of access to health care and social services within this area. The Community Needs Index (CNI) developed by the New York State Department of Health, AIDS Institute, to help in identifying and directing health care and prevention services to communities most in need, ranked Crown Heights as "high need." Moreover, all zip codes in the Crown Heights area ranked in the top 10 of the CNI score out of 37 zip codes in the borough of Brooklyn (Community Needs Index, New York State Department of Health AIDS Institute, December, 2000).

A major determinant in the spread of HIV in the Caribbean community is the high rates of Sexually Transmitted Diseases (STDs) among the adult population. While the rate of STDs in New York City is reported to have decreased 14% from 1998 to 1999, the rates of gonorrhea and chlamydia increased by 14% and 22% respectively in the Crown Heights area. The New York City Department of Health reported that Crown Heights ranked first in Brooklyn for rates of gonorrhea, chlamydia and primary and secondary syphilis. Overall, Crown Heights ranked third for gonorrhea, sixth for chlamydia and eleventh for primary and secondary syphilis in New York City. These rates of STDs cannot be divorced from the prevailing sexual behavior and practices within this community (New York City Department of Health 1998-99 STD Surveillance Data).

Key socio-structural factors such as poverty, homophobia and racism have been associated with high-risk sexual behavior among gay and bisexual men, especially those of color (Ramirez-Valles, 2002). Black men in the City of New York are more likely to die from AIDS than white and Latino men. Black men in the City of New York, between the ages of 15 and 22 years who have sex with men, were classified by The Centers for Disease Control and Prevention (CDC) as a high-risk group. The infection rate among this group was 5%.

The spread of HIV/AIDS in the population of New York City is complex. According to Johnson (2000), "one common thread is how closely racism, poverty, low self-esteem, and hopelessness are interwoven into the AIDS crisis in the black community. If people don't believe a positive future awaits, how motivated will they be to protect themselves or their partners?" (p. 3). The extent of the spread of HIV/AIDS in the Caribbean population of New York is not accidental. According to Wright (2000), "as early as 1983, African Americans accounted for 26% of national AIDS cases. In New York State African Americans have accounted for at least a third of reported AIDS cases yearly since 1982" (p. 2).

In a policy environment where HIV/AIDS policy response was targeted at injection-drug users and gay men, there was no reason for the black community to feel threatened by the spread of the disease. In particular, in the Caribbean immigrant community where injection-drug use is low or non-existent and where homosexuality is frowned upon there was no anxiety about the disease and public policy efforts were not sufficiently targeted at this community. This was a particularly imprudent approach by policymakers to HIV/AIDS given established knowledge that the black community remains susceptible to a host of health problems whether it is diabetes, asthma or heart disease.

SOCIO-STRUCTURAL FACTORS AND HIV/AIDS

Socio-structural factors within societies play a key role in determining patterns of behavior as well as a community's ability to access health care and other resources. For the Caribbean population socio-structural barriers are generally encountered in their attempts to migrate and to settle in a new place. Migration patterns among Caribbean immigrants may also contribute to the increase of the HIV rate. For example, Caribbean families often do not migrate as a unit. More commonly, one of the adults migrates first leaving the children and the other adult behind. The expectation is that they will be reunited once the adult who migrated has established him or herself in the new country. Long periods of separation which usually accompany migration sometimes result in situations where one or both of these individuals become involved in temporary relationships until they are reunited with their spouses or steady partners.

Not all Caribbean migrants move away for extended periods. In many cases immigrants use a revolving door strategy in which they might visit other countries, such as the United States, and work for short periods of time before returning to the Caribbean. Whether people migrate for long or short periods of time, engagement in sexual activity during periods of separation, particularly with partners whose sexual history is unknown or suspect, might result in the transmission of the HIV virus.

The spread of HIV/AIDS as evidenced by the increase in HIV seroprevalence among Haitians living in the Bateyes of the Dominican Republic is a good example of how commonly HIV is transmitted among migrant groups. HIV rates among these workers doubled from 7% in 1991 to 15% in 1997. A high rate of HIV seroprevalence has also been found to be present among males working in the mining industry in Guyana. Some 6% of these workers, who were migrants from the coastal area to the hinterland of Guyana, were found by the Centers for Disease Control and Prevention (CDC) to be HIV positive (CAREC, 2001).

A major catalyst of HIV/AIDS in the black population and by extension, the Caribbean population in New York City, is the criminal justice system. Black men, without steady living wages, provide a continuous clientele for the criminal justice system. Yet, it is in the confines of prisons that many men contract HIV/AIDS because of the lack of access to condoms and the failure to educate prisoners about the dangers of HIV/AIDS.

Estimates of the HIV-positive population in statewide prisons across the United States were reported by the United States Department of Justice as 7,500 at the end of 1997. In a criminal justice system that housed one in 31 Black men and one in 79 Latino men in 1997, a large subsection of Caribbean men are at risk of contracting HIV/AIDS while serving prison time. New York State's prison population comprised 48% Black and 45% Latino compared with 7% of Whites (Wright, 2000). The impact of the release of prisoners from the New York State prisons back into the minority neighborhoods creates concern for advocates in these communities. According to Wright (2000), "What happens when ex-offenders transition from prison back to the block is an area of great concern for those working to stem HIV's spread in the black communities. It's unclear whether more people are getting infected while in jail, or if they are just finding out about their infections while locked up." Outreach workers in New York City have focused on educating persons leaving prisons and encouraging them to engage in safe sexual practices.

Disdain of homosexual behavior among the Caribbean population has caused many gay men to engage in sexual activities secretly while also engaging in sexual relations with women to hide their homosexual activities. Continued discrimination towards homosexuals and people living with HIV/AIDS also results in low use of testing, and thereby an increase in risky sexual behavior (Ramirez-Valles, 2002). These patterns of behavior accelerate the transmission of HIV among the Caribbean population both in the countries of origin and abroad.

Misperceptions persist among the Caribbean population about the nature and cause of HIV/AIDS. Many use a religious perspective to apportion blame to victims for "lewd" behavior that results in punishment through this afflic-tion. This approach to the problem of HIV/AIDS, in the context of the lives of the Caribbean population, is as inhumane as it is misguided. A more sensitive and potentially effective response to HIV/AIDS is to consider the disease as a developmental problem that requires governmental priority and a multi-sec-toral response.

The crisis of HIV/AIDS in the black population in the city of New York is often laid at the altar of the black churches. Advocates view the perceived in-action of the black churches as a result of the tensions that exist in religious ideology between abstinence and prevention. For decades, the thinking re-mained fixed within black churches that the HIV virus was prevalent among gay men, a group not considered by many to be prominent in the membership of churches, therefore there was no reason to worry about HIV/AIDS in their church congregations. What now appears to be a virulent spread of the disease among the membership of black churches, has forced many black churches to find ways to respond to the disease.

ATTITUDES TOWARD HIV/AIDS IN CARIBBEAN SOCIETIES

Fear and denial among segments of Caribbean society trigger an increase in the number of cases of HIV/AIDS. The continued social stigma and discrimi-nation toward HIV infected persons also continue to drive the epidemic under-ground. Many victims, while in denial of their HIV positive status, often refrain from seeking medical assistance but continue to have unprotected sex with other partners thereby transmitting the disease to others.

Efforts to educate the Caribbean population about HIV/AIDS have failed to destroy the myths or changed prevailing misperceptions about the disease. A recent report on the national knowledge, attitudes, behavior and practices among the Jamaican population showed that despite the sample population's knowledge and awareness of the various prevention methods, strong mythical beliefs regarding HIV/AIDS remained prominent among the Jamaican popu-lation (Jamaica Aids Support, 2002). Based on their misguided beliefs, more than half of the sample population–93% of men and 86% of women who self-reported as sexually active–was convinced that they stood "no chance" of contracting the HIV virus. These misconceptions combined with the low approval rate of condom use among males and females have been a major factor in the increase and spread of HIV/AIDS in Jamaica as well as across the Caribbean community.

Ambiguity in the messages shared across segments of the Caribbean population towards sex promotes secretive and potentially dangerous sexual encounters among couples. Young girls who are taught to avoid sexual encounters until marriage secretly engage in sexual relations, often with older men who can provide some form of economic support. According to Stuart (2000), the Caribbean male promiscuous lifestyle is reinforced by cultural beliefs that value infidelity among men who engage in concurrent or serial relationships regardless of their marital status. Such behavior is rewarded with heroic approval among male peers and often in the wider society. However, this behavior, combined with problems of male dominance, passive submission of many Caribbean women to men's sexual advances and subsequent unprotected sexual intercourse, place women at risk of contracting HIV even when they are faithful to their partners.

Among the Caribbean population there is little evidence of sustained mutual fidelity, partner reduction, engagement in safe sexual behavior, and the practice of alternatives to penetrative sex in the heterosexual Caribbean community (Camara, 2000). Failure to change patterns of behavior despite knowledge of the devastating impact of HIV/AIDS suggests that the challenge in changing behavior is enormous. The need for a model of intervention that projects responsible behavior seems most appropriate for the Caribbean population.

IMPLICATIONS FOR AN INTERVENTION MODEL IN THE CARIBBEAN POPULATION

Although Caribbean family relations are generally organized around an extended family system, fear and stigmatization related to HIV/AIDS often change these tightly knit relationships. Once an individual's diagnosis is known there is generally widespread speculation about the method of transmission. The worst fears are often that a female victim might have been unfaithful to her partner or a male victim had engaged in homosexual activities. The infected person is immediately made to feel like an outcast as the community and in some cases family members begin to distance themselves from the victim. Feelings of isolation and stigmatization often cause the infected person to withdraw socially and emotionally at a time when they most need the support of loved ones. Among the immigrant Caribbean population, HIV infected persons often become fearful that news of their diagnosis will reach their family members in their home countries, bringing dishonor upon the family. It, therefore, becomes natural for individuals diagnosed with HIV/AIDS to keep their diagnoses private, thereby unwittingly pushing the epidemic underground.

Health economists in the Caribbean expect the impact of HIV/AIDS on the Caribbean population and economy to be severe. Similar predictions are being made in the United States where groups at the local level, such as the Caribbean Women's Health Association in Brooklyn, New York, have tackled the problem of HIV/AIDS as a multifaceted community problem. The Association's efforts to address the problem of HIV/AIDS are part and parcel of an holistic policy approach that addresses problems of immigration, housing, employment and the general well-being of the Caribbean community.

Targeted responses like that of the Caribbean Women's Health Association are urgently needed to stop the spread of HIV from reducing the economically active Caribbean population. If HIV continues to spread among the Caribbean population, it is bound to reduce the number of workers at home and abroad that are needed to boost the Gross Domestic Product of the Caribbean region. Reduction in the number of Caribbean workers employed in the United States labor force will potentially reduce the level of remittances these workers send back to their home countries. These remittances are relied upon heavily by Caribbean economies to meet the burden of external debts as well as to fund development of these economies. Unless checked soon, Caribbean economies could soon begin to experience negative growth. Such growth characterized by a fall in the level of the Gross Domestic Product and eventually, a fall in the level of domestic savings, will undermine these economies' potential to generate the income needed by governments to purchase, among other things, the anti-retroviral drugs that HIV/AIDS victims need.

Policymakers around the world are searching for models of intervention that would effectively change the patterns of behavior among populations considered as high-risk for contracting HIV/AIDS. It has now been established that to do nothing is not an option for governments in the face of the increasing number of deaths among the vulnerable, voiceless and powerless poor around the world. An effective intervention model must engage with new policies and paradigms that educate the public and reduce the stigma of HIV/AIDS.

Many interventions models are based on Social Cognitive Theory which establishes that change in behavior stems from expectations that the action of an individual can bring about specific outcomes. However, because change does not occur on its own, there must be a process or processes through which the change might occur. At the level of the individual, family and community, the model of community involvement promises to be efficacious with the Caribbean population (Ramirez-Valles, 2002). As a model that has successfully promoted self-efficacy in the use of condoms in other populations it can be beneficial in promoting self-efficacy among the Caribbean population. The model proposes changing patterns of risky behavior through listening to and observing others. This model is applicable to service programs developed to serve victims of HIV/AIDS, their families and loved ones as well as community groups. By getting involved in community work targeted to educate the public about HIV/AIDS and to support victims of HIV/AIDS, individuals will be able to share their experiences, learn from others and from educators about safer sex and enjoy mutual emotional support. Such community involvement builds a sense of camaraderie that reduces the feelings of alienation that many victims of HIV/AIDS might feel once they are diagnosed with HIV/AIDS.

Effective response to HIV/AIDS in the Caribbean community must address the reality that HIV/AIDS can no longer be trivialized. The hopelessness that is felt by many victims because of this disease could be mitigated if communities are less judgmental and more accepting of those who are infected with the virus. Less focus on the means of contracting HIV and more attention to the needs of HIV victims is desperately needed to provide the care and support that victims require. The ultimate goal must be to change patterns of behavior through ongoing public education about HIV/AIDS. A shared responsibility for the well-being of the entire population remains the best way of combating HIV/AIDS, particularly among those in the community that are most vulnerable and powerless.

REFERENCES

AIDS New York City Surveillance Update (First Quarter, June 2000). NYC Office of AIDS Surveillance: NYC Department of Health, NY: Author.

Ajzen, I., & Fishbein, M. (1980). *Understanding attitudes and predicting social behavior*. Englewood Cliffs, NJ: Prentice Hall.

Bandura, A. (1977). *A social learning theory*. Englewood Cliffs, NJ: Prentice Hall.

Becker, M.H. (1974). The Health Belief Model and personal health behavior. *Health Education Monographs*, 2, 324-508.

Becker, M.H. (1988). AIDS and behavior change. *Public Health Reviews*, 16, 1-11.

Bryan A.T. The Caribbean's Worst Plague: HIV/AIDS. North-South Center Update. Retrieved at *http://www.miami.edu/nsc/publications/newsupdates/Update51.html* (February 6, 2002).

Camara, B. (2000). An overview of the AIDS/HIV situation in the Caribbean. In Howe, Glenford & Cobley, Alan (Ed.), *The Caribbean AIDS epidemic*. Jamaica: University of the West Indies Press.

Camara, B. Twenty years of HIV/AIDS Epidemic in the Caribbean–A Summary. Powerpoint presentation. Retrieved at *http://www.carec.org/pdf/20years-aids-Caribbean.pdf*

Caribbean Epidemiology Centre (CAREC) (2001). CAREC Strategic Plan for the Prevention and Control of the HIV/AIDS Epidemic in the Caribbean: 2001-2005. Port of Spain, Trinidad: *CAREC/PAHO/WHO.*

Carr R. *Stigmas, Coping and gender: A study of HIV+ Jamaicans, Race, class and gender* (in press)

City of New York Office of Management and Budget, Department of City Planning. (Fiscal Year 2001). *Community District needs:* Brooklyn, NY: Author.

Department of Health and Human Services (2001). *HIV/AIDS Survelliance Report. U.S. HIV and AIDS cases reported through June 2001, 13*(1). CDC: Atlanta, GA.

Department of Health and Human Services (2000). *HIV/AIDS Survelliance Report. U.S. HIV and AIDS cases reported through December 2000, 13*(1). CDC: Atlanta, GA.

Figueroa, J.P. (2001) Health trends in Jamaica: Significant progress and a Vision for the 21st century *West Indian Med J* 2001:50 (Suppl. 4) 15-22.

Francis, Claudette (2000). The Psychosocial dynamic of the AIDS epidemic in the Caribbean. In Howe, Glenford & Cobley, Alan (Ed.), *The Caribbean AIDS epidemic.* Jamaica: University of the West Indies Press.

Gray, M. (1997). African Americans. In Phillco, J. & Brisbane, F.L (Eds.), *Cultural competence in substance abuse prevention.* NASW Press; Washington DC.

HIV/AIDS Surveillance Report (2000). *US HIV/AIDS cases reported through June 2000.* U.S. Department of Health and Human Services/Public Health Service/Center for Disease Control and Prevention (Year-end-Edition, Vol. 10, No. 1). Atlanta, GA: Author.

Hope Enterprises Ltd. *Report of the National Knowledges, Attitudes, Behaviour and Practices Survey Year 2000,* Kingston, Jamaica, 2001.

Howe, Glenford & Cobley, Alan (2000). *The Caribbean AIDS epidemic.* Jamaica: University of the West Indies Press.

Jamaica AIDS Support (2002). The HIV/AIDS External Environment. Retrieved from *http://www.jamaicasidssupport.com/strategicplan/externalenv.htm*

Johnson, K. (June 28-July 4, 2000). Aids and Black New Yorkers. The Tuskegee Effect. For Blacks, a 28-year old study is one of many barriers to HIV prevention. Retrieved from: *http://www.villagevoice.com/issues/0026/johnson.php*

Marquez, P. Fighting AIDS in the Caribbean. *En breve.* June 2002. Vol. No. 4.

New York City Department of Health (2000). *1998-1999 STD Surveillance data by New York City neighborhood,* NY: Author.

New York State Department of Health, AIDS Institute (December 2000). *Community Needs Index (CNI).* Albany NY: Author

Nicholls, S. et al. *Modelling the macroeconomic impact of HIV/AIDS in the English-speaking Caribbean: The case of Trinidad and Tobago and Jamaica.* Caribbean Epidemology Centre/University of the West Indies/PAHO/WHO.

Ramsammy, L. (2003) *Caribbean response to HIV/AIDS.* Ministry of Health, Guyana

Ramirez-Valles, J. (2002). The protective effects of community involvement for HIV risk behavior: A conceptual framework. *Health Education Research, Theory and Practice.* Vol. 17. No. 4, 389-403.

Stuart, Sheila (2000). The reproductive health challenge: Women and AIDS in the Caribbean. In Howe, Glenford and Cobley, Alan (Ed.), *The Caribbean AIDS epidemic.* Jamaica: University of the West Indies Press.

TransAfrica Forum Issue Brief. AIDS in the Caribbean. September 2002.

UNAIDS, "Fact Sheet: HIV/AIDS in the Caribbean" February 2001. Retrieved from *http://www.unaids.org/fact_sheets/files/Caribbean_Eng.doc* (July 23, 2001).

World Bank Group (2003). *Combating HIV/AIDS in the Caribbean through a comprehensive, multisectoral approach.*

Wright, K. (July 5-11, 2000). AIDS and Black New Yorkers. Double Jeopardy. In New York State Blacks Rank Highest Among HIV-positive Inmates. Retrieved from *http://www.villagevoice.com/issues/0027/wright.php*

Yilma, Marda (2001). 2001 North Crown Heights AIDS profile. *Brooklyn AIDS Task Force Community Resources, NY.*

Working with Caribbean Immigrants After the World Trade Center Tragedy: A Challenge for Social Work Practice

Lear Matthews

SUMMARY. Caribbean immigrants were among those transfixed by the destruction and human suffering caused by the World Trade Center tragedy. An emergent cliché is that life will never be the same after September 11th. This study explores the issues that impact the health and well-being of English-speaking Caribbean immigrants and challenges social workers to reassess their intervention with immigrant populations in the Post 9/11 era. *[Article copies available for a fee from The Haworth Document Delivery Service: 1-800-HAWORTH. E-mail address: <docdelivery@haworthpress.com> Website: <http://www.HaworthPress.com> © 2004 by The Haworth Press, Inc. All rights reserved.]*

KEYWORDS. Caribbean immigrants, World Trade Center tragedy, social work

INTRODUCTION

Caribbean immigrants were among those transfixed by the destruction and human suffering caused by the World Trade Center tragedy of September

---

Lear Matthews, DSW, is affiliated with SUNY Empire State College.

[Haworth co-indexing entry note]: "Working with Caribbean Immigrants After the World Trade Center Tragedy: A Challenge for Social Work Practice." Matthews, Lear. Co-published simultaneously in *Journal of Immigrant & Refugee Services* (The Haworth Social Work Practice Press, an imprint of The Haworth Press, Inc.) Vol. 2, No. 3/4, 2004, pp. 69-82; and: *The Health and Well-Being of Caribbean Immigrants in the United States* (ed: Annette M. Mahoney) The Haworth Social Work Practice Press, an imprint of The Haworth Press, Inc., 2004, pp. 69-82. Single or multiple copies of this article are available for a fee from The Haworth Document Delivery Service [1-800-HAWORTH, 9:00 a.m. - 5:00 p.m. (EST). E-mail address: docdelivery@haworthpress.com].

69

11th, 2001 in New York City, where a substantive segment of the population is foreign-born. Coupled with the continuous threat of terrorism, the disaster gave rise to an admixture of emotional and political reverberations which have affected the well-being of native-born Americans, and immigrants alike. An emergent cliché is that life will never be the same after September 11th. But what does this mean for thousands of immigrants in the United States? This study explores the issues and problems that impact the lives of English-speaking Caribbean immigrants following the tragedy, and challenges social workers to reassess their intervention with immigrant populations in the post 9/11 era.

Farkas, Duffett and Johnson (2003) note that the disaster and its aftermath appear to have escalated the skepticism of the American public about the country's openness to immigration. Yet, people who were killed, traumatized or otherwise affected were of myriad ethnicities, occupations and nationalities. Corzine (2003, p. 28) suggests, "The terrorists made no distinction between American citizens and aliens killed in the attack, and we should not set aside the heroism of those aliens who died, and the terrible impact on their families." *The Immigrant's Journal* (2001) reported that about 40% of lives lost were from countries other than the United States, including scores from the Caribbean region. More than sixty families from English-speaking Caribbean nations such as Jamaica, Barbados, Guyana, Trinidad and Tobago, Antigua, Grenada, Dominica, the Bahamas and St. Lucia were left to mourn the deaths of relatives (Caribbean Losses, 2002). Furthermore, it is estimated that a number of the undocumented who were missing, were Caribbean-American laborers whose families were not eligible for survivor benefits, among them delivery persons, messengers and others doing temporary, menial jobs.

THE PROBLEM:
SOCIAL ISSUES AND POLICY CHANGES

Effective social work intervention could be determined by how well practitioners are grounded in the knowledge of contemporary social issues and events that impact the lives of potential clientele. Many in the immigrant community appear to be suffering in silence while facing a number of obstacles in the aftermath of September 11th. Demanding an investigation into the treatment of immigrants since the September 11th tragedy, a group of public officials in New York City argued that, immigrant communities have been unreasonably targeted by legal authorities and many of their needs have been ignored (Cheng, 2002). In the wake of the attack, friends and relatives of missing undocumented immigrants from the Caribbean who are themselves undocumented were reluctant to notify the authorities (Caribbean Losses, 2002), fearing detention and possible deportation. An example of the morass of uncertainty in which Caribbean immigrants found themselves, is the case of a Guyanese immigrant who was afraid to report his undocumented son missing in the rubble. One month later, with some trepidation he obtained a death certificate for his son upon hearing a public official's promise that there will be "no repercussions for reporting undocumented workers lost in the disaster" (Ross and Hutchinson, 2003, p. 14). A young Trinidadian woman, the last of four persons to be found alive in the rubble of the collapsed site, is another case in point. As an unauthorized worker in the World Trade Center on the day of the disaster, it is unlikely that she and others in that situation would be deported (Cloud, 2002). However, it is not clear whether the government's policy on such issues was adequately publicized through organizations in immigrant communities.

In his assessment of post 9/11 experiences of Caribbean immigrants, Andrew Lam (2003, p. 12) concludes, "Since that terrible day of September 11, 2001, the immigrant's hold on American soil has become increasingly tenuous, if not outright threatened. In the name of protection and security, immigrants' rights are being eroded. . . . These days an immigrant can lose his job because he is not yet a U.S. citizen, and if he speaks his opinion, he can very well be fired."

The newly created Department of Homeland Security (DHS, 2003) has led to several policies and procedural changes, which include a "process that gives the government knowledge of every immigrant's current status and location" (King, 2003, p. 19). For instance, immigrants (including Green Card holders) who fail to report a change of address within two weeks, could be arrested and deported. City and state police are authorized to enforce federal immigration laws and many English-speaking Caribbean immigrants are among those subjected to unusual scrutiny and surveillance by U.S. immigration authorities, following reports of suspected links to terrorist organizations (Rodney, 2003).

Referring to the experience of Caribbean immigrants, King (2003, p. 6) notes that "the heightened attacks on immigrants are nothing but very discriminating and craving for enhanced and insidious knowledge of aliens' whereabouts is the most disturbing legacy of 9/11." These governmental reforms may be a necessary deterrent against further terrorism, but as Hassan (2003) warns, this could lead to an undermining of community trust and draining of resources.

East Indians from the English-speaking Caribbean living in the United States have been subjected to discriminatory acts, due to their physical resemblance to Middle Eastern immigrants. The recently publicized harassment and killings of Caribbean immigrants in New York City and Florida were described as violence against "terrorists" and "patriotic assassinations" by individuals who allegedly wanted revenge for the September 11 attacks (Grace, 2003; Ali, 2003). Writing in the *New York Times*, Sterngold (2001) refers to the negative impact of the government's attitude of suspicion with regards to certain immigrants, creating an atmosphere that could cause some of those who have had political problems in their home country and the undocumented, to be driven further underground.

The continuous state of terrorist alert is likely to be used as justification for detention and deportation proceedings against immigrants in general, a situation which has created numerous social, political and psychological difficulties. There has been some concern among Caribbean immigrant service providers about the "distressing number of immigrants deported, especially since the 9/11 terrorist attacks" (King, 2003, p. 7). As a result of deportations, homes will be left without breadwinners, children without fathers, while in the Caribbean it appears as though no adequate provision is made for the reintegration of deportees, some of whom have been blamed for the increase in criminal activity there. Anticipated fear of international travel, job loss and stricter immigration laws (Rodney, 2003), have led to the belief that sending remittances to the home country will become a complex and arduous task. However, Hernandez (2003) found that some immigrants have actually increased the amount of remittances they send to the home country, "in case they lose their jobs in the United States or are deported" (p. 4B).

Caribbean immigrants are subjected to both the benefits and challenges of "minority communities" in the U.S. Kendall Stewart, a Caribbean-born Council member, noted that as a result of the more than 160,000 jobs lost in New York since September 11th, coupled with the huge taxpayers' share of paying for the war in Iraq, many immigrants could face "a very bleak and depressing future" (Stewart, 2003). Indeed such conditions will make the American dream quite elusive for some.

It is important that social workers working with English-speaking Caribbean immigrants and those planning to migrate to the United States understand the implications of the above-mentioned sociological and policy issues and develop strategies of intervention in concert with other helping professionals, to alleviate social and psychosocial difficulties associated with such problems.

Psychological Factors

It is inevitable that emotional health problems would emerge as a result of an event such as the September 11th tragedy. Undoubtedly, any trauma of this magnitude shatters commonly held beliefs about safety and security of one's adopted country, especially for those immigrants from nations with a spiraling crime rate or where there is political unrest. Among Caribbean and other immigrant groups, the stress created by draconian immigration laws has further exacerbated feelings of confusion, helplessness and vulnerability, particularly among the undocumented and those awaiting adjustment of immigrant status, groups that tend not to readily reach out for assistance. But documented residents are also worried, as Hernandez (2003, p. B4) notes: "Since September 11, even legal immigrants have been afraid to return to their home countries because they fear complications when they try to reenter the United States. Instead of spending money on plane tickets . . . they send the money home." One wonders whether Caribbean immigrants experience inner conflict over their loyalties to their adopted country that also discriminates against them.

How well people cope with the effects of a disaster of this magnitude, depends on a number of factors including personal resilience, i.e., the capacity to return to a perceived state of normalcy, and the social and political climate. It is not known how many people suffered from Post Traumatic Stress Disorder in the wake of the disaster, but the onset of critical incident stress, i.e., the worrying produced by "any sudden or unexpected traumatic event that affects people's emotional lives, feelings of safety, and ability to cope" was to be expected (CISD, 2001). Gerow (1997) notes that distressing symptoms arise in the aftermath of such a traumatic occurrence among those who have "experienced or witnessed . . . an event that involves actual or threatened death or serious injury and the response involves intense fear and helplessness." Reportedly, over 60% of households in New York City experienced some level of distress among family members, including a significant number of children (Schlenger, 2002). These figures undoubtedly include Caribbean immigrants, since mental hygiene treatment facilities in immigrant communities also reported increase in referrals, and relapses among their clients (O. Sheppard, psychiatric social worker, personal communication, March 19, 2003).

Some immigrants, already feeling detached due to the migration experience or marginalized because of their status, could be further alienated in the aftermath of the disaster. Others may attempt to form closer alliances with American social institutions to demonstrate their loyalty to their adopted country or as a defense against hostilities toward them. It is against this backdrop, that the post-9/11 experiences of English-speaking Caribbean immigrants and the role of social work are examined.

METHOD

A qualitative, exploratory design was used for the study. Qualitative social work research helps to demonstrate the ways in which people interpret events that affect their lives and view events from different perspectives (Neuman, 2003). The goal of the study is to examine the impact of the World Trade Center tragedy on the social and psychological well-being of English-speaking Caribbean immigrants. A second objective is to identify the role of social work in developing strategies for responding to the tragedy-related difficulties. Data collection was in the form of questionnaires, which were used to gain an in-depth understanding of the issues and problems presented by immigrants and the experiences of social workers, who worked with this population after the World Trade Center tragedy.

Fifty questionnaires were sent out to social workers and forty-one (41) were returned completed. This accounted for a response rate of 80%. The selection of respondents was based on their willingness to participate in the study and their access to Caribbean immigrants. They vary in gender, years of employment and ethnic background, and their primary responsibilities were mental hygiene counseling and case management. The data were first organized in accordance with the methodology, i.e., questionnaires, followed by the description of patterns, themes and experiences of the respondents. Of importance was the development of systematic categories, which were determined by "recurring regularities" in the data (Patton, 1989).

FINDINGS

Most of the respondents worked at the Bedford Stuyvesant Community Mental Health Center and The Visiting Nurses Services, located in New York City, in communities with a large English-speaking Caribbean immigrant population. Ethnically, the sample included twenty-six Caribbean-Americans, six African-Americans, five Caucasians and four Latinos. Data for the study were acquired from the social workers' interviews and intervention with clients. The practitioners' observations and experience with the wider English-speaking Caribbean community after the tragedy were also reported. Thirty-two of them provided direct counseling and case management services to Caribbean immigrants on issues relating to the tragedy and nine (9) did not provide such services. The concerns of the practitioners and their clients were grouped into three categories, (1) post 9/11 social/psychological problems; (2) coping strategies; and (3) the role of social work in alleviating the problems. The problems or complaints centered on safety and security issues; psychological stress; and hardship/restrictions from post 9/11 immigration policies.

Safety and Psychological Stress

Twenty-seven (27) respondents reported on feelings of insecurity, ambivalence or fear (including fear of flying to the Caribbean to visit family members, and deportation) among their clients, as well as the wider English-speaking Caribbean population. The following were reported: *I feel isolated and concerned about deportation, not receiving medical or health benefits; At one time America was a place where one could earn money, live well and return to the Caribbean feeling secure . . . this has changed since 9/11; I am afraid of losing my job and not being eligible for compensation; Why are we involved in a fight with the U.S. government when we have nothing to do with it; I'm afraid of being called un-American and treated by Americans as mistrusted foreigners; afraid of being confused with Arabs, since many Caribbeans look Arabic; more discrimination against accented immigrants; I have a student's visa and am afraid to travel to the Caribbean for my cousin's funeral; I am concerned for the safety of relatives living in the U.S. after September 11th.* While some said that they were afraid of being deported because of their immigration status, others wished to return to the Caribbean to visit relatives, but were afraid to fly.

The majority of the respondents (86%) expressed variants of psychological stress after the World Trade Center tragedy, much of it characterized by anxiety and fear regarding their social, economic and physical well-being. In this regard, responses included: *the client cried throughout the session and was afraid to go to work; many immigrants are still traumatized by the idea of taking a flight to the Caribbean.* Four clients were diagnosed with Post Traumatic Stress Disorder. *I feel stressed out when riding the subway,* reported one client, while others stated that they worry all the time, but sometimes *get very angry.* The social workers reported that several months after the tragedy, a significant number of Caribbean immigrants were treated for depression, anxiety and sleep difficulties. Presenting problems include feelings of fear, sadness, loss, and grief relating to loss of relatives or friends. *Since September 11th, I feel uncertain, helpless,* reported one individual and another developed a pinched nerve and was very distressed, since he could not afford the doctor's fee. One client was tearful because he worried about taking care of his family after the WTC tragedy, and several of them were concerned about their relatives in the Caribbean.

Owing to the incredible nature of the attacks, some immigrants referred to a sort of displacement or disorientation which felt as if they were *in a different place.* Uncertainty about the future and concerns about other Caribbean immigrants being racially profiled as terrorists were also common themes. The social workers reported that the presenting problem of a significant number of their clients (74%), including the elderly, centered on thoughts, feelings and *worrying* about September 11th. Because many of the elderly immigrants are homebound, they were *glued to the TV for extended periods after the attacks*, reported one respondent, and were bombarded with *images of an invasion that made them very depressed*. An added concern of the elderly was the fear of losing the service of caregivers and other resources to lost jobs and reduced benefits. One elderly immigrant asked, *what would happen to us now? I may be better off in my own country*.

Impact of Changing Immigration Laws

Central to the well-being of immigrants in the United States, following the World Trade Center tragedy, are the repercussions from changes in immigration laws. Apart from highlighting the impact of post-9/11 immigration policy on Caribbean immigrants, the data presented the opportunity to examine emerging issues relating to social workers' knowledge of changing immigration procedures and skill in disaster counseling. Fifty percent (21) of the social workers reported that they were not aware of any changes in U.S. immigration policy that would affect Caribbean or other immigrants; fifteen stated that they were knowledgeable of such changes; while four did not respond.

Those who had some knowledge of the changes in immigration policy had either heard about the USA PATRIOT ACT (Uniting and Strengthening America by Providing Appropriate Tools Required to Intercept and Obstruct Terrorism) or were aware of visa or other travel restrictions instituted by the Homeland Security Department. Among the responses reported were: *I think that Caribbean immigrants are afraid that if they visit their homeland, they may face great obstacles in reentering the U.S.; Some immigrants decided to abdicate themselves from completing the application for U.S. entry; I am concerned that the INS* (Immigration and Naturalization Service) *will decrease the number of people entering the country and people will be deported for minor infractions; My brother's student visa was cancelled when he returned home to visit; I anticipate a decrease in resources for immigrants*.

Others cited increased racial profiling of Caribbean and other immigrants of color, being scrutinized, increased surveillance, and extended delays in the visa application process since 9/11. As noted by one respondent, *Many English-speaking Caribbean immigrants of East Indian heritage look middle-eastern and when they travel, they are routinely stopped and questioned at airports, causing much anxiety, embarrassment and frustration*. To some extent, confidence in the host society's accommodation of immigrants has been diluted. *Some Caribbean immigrants I know think that it is no longer a plus to have an American passport when traveling overseas because of the attitude of Americans and America*, stated one respondent and others wondered about the overall effect on their immigration status since the alleged terrorists were immigrants.

Coping Strategies

Ways of coping with the above-mentioned social and psychological stresses and knowledge of coping strategies used by immigrants are of major interest in this study. Three methods of coping were identified by the respondents, namely: reaching out to family and friends; increased involvement in religious institutions; community services (including counseling), and in some instances, a combination of these. There were reports of individuals' increased alcohol consumption and sexual activity as a way of coping. One individual talked about remigrating to the Caribbean and another decided to keep a low profile and not to venture out of his *ethnic community*.

The success of immigrants' methods of coping in the aftermath of the tragedy is examined within the context of social workers' perception of the complexities of the situation and intervention. Twenty-six (26) respondents reported that they thought the resources used for coping (family and peers, church and counseling) were effective; nine (9) reported that these methods were not effective; and six (6) did not know or did not respond. Although some individuals did not follow through with referrals for professional help, because they had no health insurance, several reported a decrease in symptoms and improved functioning as a result of counseling. However, only four (4) social workers had received specialized training in disaster counseling.

The social workers in this study viewed themselves as part of an interdisciplinary team that responded to those in need including immigrants, in the wake of the disaster. They expressed concern for the *unequal treatment when it comes to helping immigrants financially and emotionally* in their efforts to recover and the lack of *expeditious intervention* in cases of bias and profiling, after September 11th. There was no support for the latter in the literature or media, but the social workers felt that they were in a vantage position to observe such occurrences.

DISCUSSION

The data provided an understanding of the experiences of social workers who worked with and observed the behaviors of English-speaking Caribbean immigrants, after the World Trade center tragedy. The study revealed a number of issues, problems and coping strategies. Emerging from the data were clear themes of concern to immigrants and practitioners. In general, the anticipated comfort and security associated with life in their adopted home have been compromised. The social workers themselves were struggling to process their own feelings with regard to the aftermath of the tragedy, while working to help others overcome fears, depression and anxiety. They were able to identify several troubling issues, exacerbated by the subjects' immigrant status (residing in the United States). Although there has been no evidence of a significant decrease in travel between the Caribbean and the United States, these immigrants appear to be more concerned about deportation or other actions that would jeopardize their residency in the United States, than the fear of in-flight or bio-terrorism per se.

The study did not reveal any correlation between immigration status (documented or undocumented) and fear of the effects of changes in immigration policy. In fact, both permanent resident immigrants and the undocumented felt that safety in the United States has been compromised by the government's implementation of anti-terrorism measures, but understood the need to be vigilant. Strong sentiment about the safety of relatives, both in the United States and the Caribbean, was expressed by immigrants, regardless of their status.

Many of the respondents were aware of the multiple restrictions in the name of Homeland Security, which potentially will not only erode civil liberties, but stymie the opportunities of immigrants. The long-term consequences of the new laws and not terrorism itself appear to be a primary source of anxiety and depression among these immigrants. In this regard Hassan (2001) warns that detention for suspected terrorism could lead to deportation for immigrant status violations, which were not hitherto associated with national security. Since 9/11, the governments of the English-speaking Caribbean countries such as Jamaica and Guyana have been known to be in rather disquieting negotiations with the United States on the issue of deportation. In addition, delays in processing citizenship and permanent residency applications will expose immigrants to deportation procedures. Furthermore, immigrants' concerns about losing their jobs, the incapacity to access services, ethnic profiling and decrease in civil rights, elucidated in this study, are certainly not unfounded as demonstrated by a recent report in which a reduction in the use of social services by immigrants, due to fear of and labeling by federal authorities, is predicted (Lam, 2003).

The coping strategies reflect the range of responses to the stress which evolved from the tragedy and anticipated long-term consequences. Family and friends as a source of help in such crises, providing support in periods of bereavement and fear, is common across nationalities and found in this study. The study also revealed that fear, anxiety and uncertainty linger among immigrants who are challenged in their daily living activities such as work, travel and family interactions. Even without the threat or consequences of terrorism, it takes time for many immigrants to inculcate the values and behaviors that are consistent with a different set of social institutions. Consequently, many of them struggle to access and negotiate adequate help from formal organizations, especially in times of crisis. Acculturative stress of the newly arrived has been exacerbated by the effects of September 11, which has also created cognitive dissonance for those immigrants, who are at various stages of perceived attainment of the American dream. This is evidenced by the continued portrayal of America as the land of the free, juxtaposed with escalating host societal restrictions.

Added to this quagmire is the nature of help-seeking behaviors of some Caribbean immigrants, characterized by non-assertiveness, a high regard for privacy and the feeling that the family can handle any problem, which often militate against facilitating assistance from agencies beyond the family group. Such attitudes may also be incongruous with coping effectively with stress from any disaster. For example, the members of a Guyanese immigrant family, who were mourning the loss of two adult children in the collapsed World Trade Center building, avoided assistance from community and city agencies. Instead, the grieving parents kept to themselves, refusing to accept professional counseling or the use of other "outside" resources (F. Ramadar, Caribbean Community Organizer, personal communication, December 10, 2001). One social worker expressed some frustration in regard to immigrants, who were *obviously distressed over the disaster, but did not want to talk about how they really feel*. It must be noted, however, that help from public agencies in the English-speaking Caribbean is usually in the form of concrete services rather than therapy or counseling, and acceptance of such assistance may be viewed as losing one's independence or being on "welfare," i.e., public assistance.

Those immigrants who stated that they were concerned about increased scrutiny and profiling were likely to be anxious, depressed or frustrated because they feel incapable of altering the host society's perception of them. As a result, some of them would be less likely to speak out on public policy issues, lest they are labeled unpatriotic or ungrateful. This in turn could strain intergroup relationships and forge insularity from non-immigrant communities.

It was interesting to find that approximately half of the social workers in the sample had little or no knowledge of significant policy changes in immigration laws and procedures since 9/11. Restrictive immigration policies would tend to result in resistance to adopting some aspects of cultural practices of the host society, but they may also foster identification with one's own ethnic/immigrant community as a "safety net." Such knowledge is fundamental in establishing a basis for social workers to identify the stressors and adaptations linked to the tragedy and its aftermath. They would also be in a fortified position to advocate for resources needed in the immigrant community, thus rendering them more effective in their intervention.

The Challenge for Social Work Practice

The role of social work in alleviating social and psychological difficulties associated with the World Trade Center tragedy and helping immigrants to develop effective coping strategies, should be informed by (1) an understanding of the cultural context of the migration experience, (2) changes in psychosocial functioning after the tragedy, and (3) the ways in which modifications in U.S. immigration policy affect the acculturation process.

Social workers must assume a sustained, leadership role in identifying and addressing the post-9/11 mental health and other needs of immigrants, within the context of consequential adjustments in the relationship between the United States and sending nations, such as those of the English-speaking Caribbean. Social workers and others in the helping professions must extend their knowledge base beyond clinical issues to include macro contingencies, such as economic and political changes, and modifications in legal systems that impact upon preparation to migrate and status adjustment (residency/citizenship) in the new society. Nevertheless, immigrants' tendency to mask clinical symptoms and their preoccupation with mundane responses and responsibilities following the disaster should be considered in assessment.

The experience of Caribbean immigrants living in the United States has generally been characterized by a process of undulating adaptation to what may be viewed as better life circumstances. But the events of September 11th, 2001 have increased the social and psychological costs of migration for some and exacerbated preexisting "transitional crises" for others. This requires planned intervention, guided by a comprehension of the needs of immigrants as they try to cope with the stress caused by the tragedy, and adjust to the new realities of post-9/11 America. Gittrich (2003, p. 12) notes that unlike natural disasters, "terror attacks tend to cause more prolonged psychological problems that cannot be addressed through quick intervention." Such an assertion is supported by this study, justifying the need for training in disaster counseling among social workers, thus helping immigrants to cope with the long-term effects of these problems. A partnership with a supportive family network, religious institutions where these obtain, and other community-based organizations would be instrumental in mobilizing immigrants. Furthermore, referrals to special programs such as the unemployment insurance program of the September 11 Fund for those who were left unemployed and uninsured after the disaster (Richardson, 2003), would be useful.

This study has provided some insight into immigrants' dilemma and need for support to alleviate the social, psychological and political obstacles that emerged since 9/11. Assistance in the effort to protect or improve their immigration status and the right to counsel if detained should be provided. Long after the tragedy, mental health providers stress the need for ongoing therapy focused on groups such as immigrants that were slow to get professional help, due to cultural or political barriers. Concomitantly, it is crucial that agencies and social workers encourage reciprocity of ideas and methods of coping used by various immigrant groups after the disaster, which would ensure mutual support and understanding.

CONCLUSION

This study has advanced the notion that English-speaking Caribbean immigrants are faced with lingering difficulties which arose from the aftermath of the World Trade Center disaster. Although the Caribbean region is in relative close proximity to the United States, the effects of the tragedy have created a social distance in vital areas of personal and social functioning.

Social workers are challenged to incorporate a repertoire of knowledge and skills that reflect a familiarity with the transforming trends and needs of the immigrant community. Indeed, human service professionals must themselves be empowered with the tools and resources to advocate for changes in government policies in accord with immigrants' rights, thus ensuring effective outcome and best practices with immigrants. Consequently, there must be ongoing educational and therapeutic support services for the practitioners, thus helping them to acquire knowledge, resources and skills in developing both emergency and long-term strategies for assisting all segments of the population in coping with a disaster of this magnitude. Collaboration between agencies serving immigrant communities and academic institutions that train and credential social workers, would facilitate this process. Mutual exchange of information, methods and experiences with immigrant populations among these entities, will enhance the effectiveness of working with them. Finally, social workers and other human service professionals should be cognizant of the benefits and detriments of immigration reform to both the host society and the immigrant community.

The experiences of a wider crosssection of social workers working with the Caribbean immigrant community cannot be accounted for here. However, it is hoped that the study has raised questions that would stimulate further research on the topic as it affects other immigrant groups, which would add to the knowledge base required for policy considerations and more effective intervention with immigrants.

REFERENCES

Ali, A. (2003) *Guyana-Born Muslim woman harassed on Florida highway*, City Desk Contact, Miami.

Caribbean Losses: World Trade Center update (2002, January) *EVERYBODY'S Caribbean Magazine*, p. 8.

Caribbean Roundup (2001) *September 11th attacks still has economic impact over Caribbean countries*, *Daily Challenge*, Thursday, December 20th.

Cheng, M. (2002) *Plea for 9/11's silent victims*, *Newsday*, Wednesday, November 20th.

CISD Information Pamphlet (2001) *Coping with a critical incident*, Maryland: International Critical Incident Stress Foundation.

Cloud, J. (2002) *A miracle's cost*, *Time*, September, 11.

Corzine, C. (2003) *Win protection for immigrant families*, *The New York CaribNews*, Vol. XIX, No.1059, February 12th.

Farkas, S., A. Duffett and J. Johnson (2003) *Now that I am here: What America's immigrants have to say about life in the U.S. today*, *American Educator*, Summer.

Gerow, J.R. *Psychology: An introduction*, New York: Longman.

Gittrich, G. (2003) *9/11 Trauma and aid in limbo: Millions unspent as relatively few seek counseling*, *Daily News*, Tuesday, May 27.

Grace, M. (2003) *Cops nab Brooklyn thrill killer*, *Daily News*, Monday, March 31st

Hassan, D. (2003) *The undocumented: Are they safe? Guyana Monitor*, July.

Hassan, D. (2001) *Unpatriotic act*, *Guyana Monitor*, December.

Hernandez, D. (2003) *With fewer dollars to go around, more are going around world*, *New York Times*, July 14th.

King, N.A. (2003) *Immigrants face greater scrutiny under new federal agency*, *Caribbean Life*, March 11th.

King, N.A. (2003) *Immigration dominates Parker's first public forum*, *Caribbean Life*, May 13, 2003.

Lam, Andrew (2003) *Is the American dream still alive? New York Liberty Star*, February 14.

National Public Radio (2003) *All things considered*, March, 30th.

Neuman, W.L. and L.W. Kreuger (2003) *Social work research methods, qualitative and quantitative approaches*, Boston: Allyn and Bacon.

Patton, M.Q. (1989) *Qualitative evaluation methods: London: Sage Publication.*

Richardson, C. (2003) *A Healthy Plan: Group aids N.Y.'s uninsured workers*, *Daily News*, Monday, August 4th.

Rodney, C. (2003) *Update from the Carib News*, WLIB Radio, *The Morning Show*, February 14th & March 26th.

Ross, B. and B. Hutchinson (2003) *Grieving father or con man? Daily News*, Tuesday, July 15th.

Schlenger, W.E. (2002) *Psychological reactions to terrorist attacks, Findings from the National Study of Americans' Reactions to September 11th*, *JAMA*, August 2002, Vol. 288, No. 5.

Sterngold, J. (2001) *Legal residency hopes of millions dashed*, *New York Times*, Sunday, October 7th.

Stewart, K. (2003) *Iraq war will be tough on poor Brooklynites pocket-books*, *New York Liberty Star*, March, 28.

The Immigrant's Journal (2001) *Immigrants lives lost in terrorist action*, OCT/NOV. *www.dhs.gov/dhspublic/themehome*

Caribbean Women's Migratory Journey: An Exploration of Their Decision-Making Process

Christiana Best-Cummings

Margery A. Gildner

SUMMARY. For Caribbean women who leave their children behind to migrate to the United States, the decision-making process is filled with pain and fraught with ambivalence. In response to open-ended questions about their migratory journey, immigrant women who migrated to New York City describe the process–from initial thoughts about leaving their home country, through the actual move, to their early days in the United States. This case study examines the painful and difficult experiences of undocumented women as they balance feelings of freedom and exhilaration with the challenges of economic survival, leaving their loved ones

Christiana Best-Cummings, MSW, CSW, is Project Manager for the Administration for Children's Services, James Satterwhite Academy in New York City, NY. Margery A. Gildner, MS, is a social work consultant in Atlanta, GA.

[Haworth co-indexing entry note]: "Caribbean Women's Migratory Journey: An Exploration of Their Decision-Making Process." Best-Cummings, Christiana and Margery A. Gildner. Co-published simultaneously in *Journal of Immigrant & Refugee Services* (The Haworth Social Work Practice Press, an imprint of The Haworth Press, Inc.) Vol. 2, No. 3/4, 2004, pp. 83-101; and: *The Health and Well-Being of Caribbean Immigrants in the United States* (ed: Annette M. Mahoney) The Haworth Social Work Practice Press, an imprint of The Haworth Press, Inc., 2004, pp. 83-101. Single or multiple copies of this article are available for a fee from The Haworth Document Delivery Service [1-800-HAWORTH, 9:00 a.m. - 5:00 p.m. (EST). E-mail address: docdelivery@haworthpress.com].

Digital Object Identifier: 10.1300/J191v2n03_06

behind, parenting children from a distance, loneliness, and adjusting to a new environment while supporting themselves and family members at home. This exploratory study identifies the significant milestones in Caribbean women's migratory journey–points at which they access internal and external resources. Practitioners will understand the process, and resources these women call upon. Both the process and the accompanying resources are vital to future work with immigrant women and their families, as well as those women considering migrating and leaving their children behind. *[Article copies available for a fee from The Haworth Document Delivery   Service: 1-800-HAWORTH.   E-mail   address: <docdelivery@ haworthpress.com> Website: <http://www.HaworthPress.com> © 2004 by The Haworth Press, Inc. All rights reserved.]*

KEYWORDS. Caribbean women, immigration, separation and loss, social work, decision-making process, internal and external resources

BACKGROUND

In the context of globalization and economic survival, immigration has brought about a dramatic demographic and economic transformation in New York City. By 1999, in New York City, 35 percent of the population was immigrants or foreign-born residents (Foner, 2001). According to the New York City Department of City Planning (1996), a large percentage of the immigrant population in New York City consists of immigrants from the Caribbean. In the 1970s, Caribbeans made up 37 percent of all immigrants; in the 1980s the number was 40 percent and in the 1990s, 33 percent. The number of people migrating from the Caribbean to New York City between 1982 and 1989 was 274,528 (New York City Department of City Planning, 1996). The exact number of *undocumented* immigrants in New York City is unknown, although the Immigration and Naturalization Service (INS) estimates that there are 540,000 undocumented immigrants throughout New York State, with the vast majority living in the City (Foner, 2001).

A gender analysis of the immigration population reveals that women are leading this trend. In the early 1990s, the gender ratio of immigrants admitted into New York City was 92 males to 100 females (Salvo and Ortiz, 1992). The gender ratio of immigrants is influenced by special provisions in the immigration law that allowed for positions in the nursing and health care field, a field with a high proportion of female workers (New York City Department of City Planning, 1996; Donato, 1992; Houston, Kramer, and Barrett, 1984). In addition, some women choose to migrate to the U.S. as a result of the "sixth preference," the nonprofessional occupational category of "live-in" domestic servants, a category that was reduced significantly by the Immigration Reform and Control Act of 1996 (Department of Justice, 1984-92 as cited by Kasinitz and Vickerman, 2001).

Immigrant women play a major role in the economy both in the United States and in their home countries. When immigrant women leave their children behind to be cared for by relatives or other adults, a practice commonly referred to as *child fostering* (Soto, 1987), it has a significant impact on the economy of the home country. Child fostering typically creates a situation in which the immigrant mother sends remittances and material goods to relatives, children and other adults who are caring for her children (Philpott, 1968 as cited in Watkins-Owens, 2001). For many developing countries, immigrant payment is one of the largest sources of foreign exchange (Kasinitz and Vickerman, 2001), because it provides relatives living at home with a higher standard of living (Foner, 2001; Kasinitz and Vickerman, 2001). Political leaders of some developing countries recognize the financial impact of their nationals living abroad, and frequently encourage these individuals to remain involved in projects that contribute in the building of their country (Basch, 2001). Some politicians even encourage their nationals to secure dual citizenship (Foner, 2001). In the United States, immigrant women are viewed by some–and, in particular, undocumented immigrants–as making a positive contribution to the economy (Gopaul-McNicol, 1993; Kaufman, as cited in Foner, et al., 2000). These women are credited for their participation in social networks, which provide job referrals and support to newcomers, and as a result give them a high rate of participation in the labor market. In large cities such as New York and Los Angeles, the growth in professional employment also creates a demand for low-wage, low-skilled jobs, which attract and are more accessible to immigrants than to native minorities (Sassen, 1988; Waldinger, 1996; Zhou, 1992; Portes and Stepick, 1993). These social networks reportedly create ethnic "niches," jobs that are saturated with the same ethnic members. At the same time, however, the social networks can lock its members into low-paying jobs associated with racial prejudice and discrimination, leading employers to select immigrant women over native blacks (Waldinger, 1996).

Rationale for the Case Study

Many studies have explored the reasons–the "why" underlying the increasing flow of immigrants from developing countries to the United States. The most common reasons identified are: economic and labor market opportunities (Salazar-Parrenas, 2001; Gopaul-McNicol, 1993); linkages with the

United States (Sassen, 1988; Ricketts, 1987); diminishing resources at home such as health care, nutrition and working conditions (Chang, 2000); and globalization (Foner, 2001). Few studies, however, explore the "how"–the process by which a woman makes the decision to migrate and leave her children behind. In addition, few studies explore the emotional and psychological trauma associated with the migratory process of women who leave their children behind. Very little is known about the challenges and struggles that women, in particular, experience *before* leaving their country of origin and their families, *during* their actual migration to the United States, or *after* they arrive and are adjusting to a new way of life while balancing the financial and emotional challenges of parenting children from a distance. Espin's (1987) model of the psychological impact of the migratory process for Latina women serves as a starting point for studying the migratory process of Caribbean women, but there is little research that examines the specific measures the woman and her family put in place to make it possible for her to leave her children and live in another country.

Espin's (1987) article, "Psychological Impact of Migration on Latinas: Implications for Psychotherapeutic Practice," examined the psychological effects of the migratory process for Latina women living in the United States. Underlying Espin's model is the issue of separation and loss for Latina immigrants, demonstrated in a type of "culture-shock" that is characterized by Latinas mourning the loss of their family members and country of origin while simultaneously adapting to their new environment. Espin's model consists of three stages beginning with the decision-making process before Latinas leave their country of origin and concluding with their adjustment to life in the United States. The authors used Espin's three stages as the foundation for developing the instrument utilized for collecting data in the study of the migratory process for Caribbean women. The goal of this study is to explore the decision-making process of the migratory process of undocumented Caribbean women, using the case study method to determine how women make the decision to migrate and leave their children behind.

Study Design

This study was designed to focus on the decision-making process of undocumented Caribbean women who migrated to New York City and left their children behind. An interview guide–based on current research and the authors' experiences and interests–was used to conduct the interviews. The interview guide consists of both structured and open-ended questions. The questions were divided into three categories: (1) initial decision concerning relocation, (2) relocation: the actual move, and (3) initial adaptation.

To identify and select participants for the study–undocumented immigrant mothers from the Caribbean region who migrated without their children–the authors used a snowball procedure. Individuals who were familiar with the Caribbean immigrant community were asked to identify Caribbean women who migrated to the United States and left their children behind. Of the 20 participants recruited, 11 of them agreed to be interviewed. The nine participants who did not agree to be interviewed told their contacts that they feared participation in the study would jeopardize their undocumented status. Some of them, however, indicated that they did not want to speak about an issue that made them sad. The women who did participate in the study had all arrived in the U.S. as undocumented workers seeking employment. These women believed that, after a brief separation, they would be able to reunite with their children either in the United States or in their country of origin.

Characteristics of the Sample

The sample consisted of 11 women from eight different countries: Grenada, Guyana, Jamaica, Trinidad, Antigua/Barbuda, St. Lucia, Panama and the Dominican Republic. At the time of migration, three women were married, three women were divorced and five were single. In addition, at the time of migration, the women ranged in ages from 24 to 30 years.

CASE STUDY:
CARIBBEAN WOMEN'S DECISION-MAKING PROCESS TO MIGRATE

The study reveals several stages that evolve from the voices of Caribbean immigrant women as they speak about their decision to migrate to the United States. The process includes the steps experienced (a) prior to migrating, (b) during the migration and (c) their initial adjustment in the United States. These steps describe patterns of behaviors that are common in the migratory process for Caribbean women.

Prior to Migrating

In this study, the initial decision-making phase for the Caribbean immigrant woman occurs prior to migrating and is comprised of a variety of steps. Although the steps are progressive in nature, they do not necessarily occur in a linear fashion–some of the six steps outlined below may occur simultaneously and be repeated. Many Caribbean women experience the "subconsciously aware" step whether or not they actually migrate to the U.S.

Step 1: Subconsciously Aware. Long before a Caribbean woman begins to think consciously of leaving her country of origin, environmental factors create subliminal thoughts of traveling overseas: "I lost my job and could not find another one for months." Frequently, there is a predecessor in the migratory process such as a friend, neighbor or family member who triggers subconscious thoughts of options or opportunities that necessitate travel: "I had a girlfriend in America who wrote me and would talk about life in America. She invited me to come visit, but I knew I couldn't because of my family."

Step 2: Consciously Aware. In the second step prior to migrating (and an integral part of the decision-making process), the woman begins to consciously or actively think of options or opportunities that require travel. Often, the woman has not shared her thoughts with anyone at this point. This stage might be triggered by factors that can be defined as situations of loss and/or trauma: job loss or unemployment, political unrest in the country of origin, divorce or separation from a spouse or partner, homelessness, or the death of a loved one. The woman can view such an incident as the "sign" she has been seeking to help her explore other options. At this point, she begins to actively think of leaving–asking herself "What If?"–but does not yet make any real plans to leave. One woman stated, "I would never have even considered moving, but then I found myself homeless with two children. I had a certain standard of living as a nurse and I was unable to build a home for my children as a single parent with no family support. I got another letter from my friend who invited me to come to NYC to work for a family she knew." One woman talked about the pain of losing her children in a divorce which "triggered" her to explore opportunities and options away from her island: She states, "An unemployed woman cannot fight for custody of her children if the father is employed and says he wants them. He had status in the community and I had no status, especially as a divorced woman." The conscious awareness phase prompts the woman to hear or see options or opportunities she had not considered before. She begins to examine what it might mean for her and her children to be separated. The practice and concept of child fostering begins to surface in her thinking. She begins to access inner resources such as her strengths, her values and resilience as she explores what she can or cannot do for herself and for her children. When an increased awareness for change occurs due to an event that is experienced as a loss or trauma, the woman often finds herself in the grief process. It is at this point that she may experience Kubler-Ross's (1969) second phase of the grieving process: *bargaining.* The increased awareness, discomfort or pain can cause the woman to bargain with herself, with God or with some higher being to give her a "sign" or assistance to make things better in her life and to make the separation from her children acceptable. One woman said, "I asked God to help me find someone good to take care of my children because I did not have any family to help. I knew if they sent me someone who could take care of my children, that was His way of saying 'Go in peace, your children would be okay.' " Another woman gave the following example of how she bargained as she experienced the consciously aware step. She stated, "It is difficult to get a visa to travel to the U.S. so I decided to make three attempts. The first two times they turned me down, but the third time I got the visa and I knew God was making it possible for me to go."

Step 3: Active Planning. The third step in the decision-making phase is active planning. At this point, the woman begins to examine various opportunities, identify options and put plans in place. When this occurs, she actively begins to gather information and talk to others about the planning and preparation for change. A woman begins to seek ways to get papers to travel to the United States or to obtain information about visa requirements or job opportunities: "I had a friend who had a family member who traveled to the United States. We would have a three-way telephone conversation that helped me hear what life was like." Another woman states, "I had to go to another country to visit a U.S embassy to get a visa." During active planning, the woman reaches out and gathers information about opportunities in the United States and specific resources to assure that her children will be taken care of in her absence. She is mobilized to take action, even in the midst of feelings of sadness or loss she may be experiencing about her current situation and the pending separation from her children. The active planning step involves examining and planning for the logistics of moving, from preparing to migrate, to the actual migration, to getting settled in the United States. A tremendous amount of energy is accessed and expended during this step. The active planning step has some characteristics comparable to the *anger* phase in Kübler-Ross's process of grief, a phase in which strong feelings are expressed in behaviors that often are intensely motivated. Some of the behaviors exhibited in the active planning step may include focused preparation, organizing, or forging ahead with a sense of strong determination: "I was so angry, my husband got custody of my children, and he remarried a month later . . . so I decided to leave. I made all the plans and three months later I left."

Step 4: Developing a Network. As information is gathered, the woman begins to initiate contact with friends and family to develop an informal network both in the country of origin and in the United States to support her move. The informal network plays a critical role in supporting and facilitating the woman's decision-making process. Support from the informal network in the U.S. can range from offering a place for the immigrant to live when she arrives, to assisting with the search for employment, to offering support in the form of financial assistance and/or socialization when the immigrant arrives: "My friend wrote and enclosed a letter from my sponsor who said she would give me a place to live, and pay me if I came to work for her." For the large number of women traveling to the United States from third-world countries the local informal network at home is essential, and just as significant, to the woman's relocation as is the support from friends in the U.S. The informal network at home often includes the person or family who will be fostering the children. Collectively, this informal network provides support to the immigrant in various ways: advice about the relocation itself and its consequences, financial support, encouragement, and at times when the extended family is not a viable option for child fostering, the informal network helps in finding child care for the immigrant's children who will be left behind. "The nurses I worked with told me how lucky I was to have the opportunity to go and work in America. I remember them telling me, 'If you don't go, I'll go.' They told me that this is an opportunity to make a better life for me and for my children. They told me that people left their children and traveled all the time. All I had to do was send for my children when I got there." Another woman recounts, "My friends told me, 'Now that you are divorced, you don't have anything to keep you here. Your kids will be fine.' They even helped pay for my airline ticket." It is these networks that encourage and support the woman to move and also keep her from turning back.

Step 5: Critical Thinking. The fifth step involves a period of time in which the woman steps back again and reexamines her reasons for leaving and her decision-making process. She weighs the pros and cons of leaving her country of origin, and weighs the pros and cons of leaving her children. This step can last from a couple of weeks to months and often continues long after the decision to travel is made and even after the woman has been living in the U.S. for a period of time. It is at this point that a woman may turn to spiritual beliefs and internal strengths to remain focused on the goal and keep her moving forward. At the same time, she may continue to weigh the pros and cons as a way of preparing herself for relocation: "I prayed and prayed for the strength and word from God about what to do."

The informal network, both in the U.S. and at home, is also instrumental in helping the woman cope with feelings of guilt and regret. Because the critical thinking stage is characterized by sadness for both the woman and her children, the immigrant reconsiders her decision to relocate. Here the woman wrestles with the perceived gains and losses, an essential component of her decision to move. Some of the most common benefits that influence the woman's decision to leave are the need to seek economic, financial and educational opportunities, for herself and her children, and/or the need to escape a trauma or to survive an earlier loss. The gains, however, are weighed against the guilt of leaving children behind: "I weighed the pros and cons for a while. It was very difficult to think of leaving my children with a stranger and not knowing what to really expect when I arrived in the U.S. I kept thinking of the long-term gains. I wanted more for my children and saw no way of getting it for them if I stayed. I was torn between leaving my children and seeing that I could never be the mother I used to be with them. I had to leave them so I can take better care of them." At this point, many women minimize the trauma and impact of separation on themselves and their children. They rationalize their decision to leave with statements like, "It will only be for a few months" or "I'm doing this for my children." These statements and beliefs are the catalysts that tip the scale for them in deciding to move forward.

Step 6: Preparation of Self and Others. Although the first five steps prepare the woman and her loved ones for relocation to the U.S., in the last of the six steps in the initial decision-making stage, the woman *actively* prepares herself and others for the move. As is true with the other steps, it is often the woman's spiritual beliefs and internal strength that keep her focused on her goal and help her proceed with the actual move. As one woman put it, "I put everything in the hands of the Lord." At this point, the informal network system also is critical in providing support and tangible assistance to the woman. The informal network in the U.S. may provide advice about packing for the trip or preparation for how to approach various immigration agents.

Preparing children for the separation depends on the age of the children, the person or family who will be fostering the child, and the mother's understanding of child development. Also important are the children's reaction to the move and the mother's ability to prepare them for an indefinite period of separation. This study revealed that immigrant mothers leaving their children behind provide minimal preparation for them around the trauma and impact of the loss and separation. One woman stated, "I didn't know what to say, they were so little that I just left." Another woman talked about the pain she experienced in trying to talk with her children: "It was too hard for me to even think about leaving them that I didn't want to talk about it." One strategy a couple of mothers used with school-age children and preteens was a series of conversations with them where the mother informs her children of the compelling reasons why she has to migrate. "I talked to my children and explained why I had to leave. I was honest with them, they understood I was leaving because I was trying to find a better life for us." But the emotional impact and trauma of the separation is rarely discussed, and because the woman views the move as a necessary choice, children understandably have little input or influence in the decision-making process.

During Migration

This stage begins with the trip to the airport in the country of origin, followed by the flight, and then the arrival and stop at Immigration. For the woman and her loved ones, this stage is fraught with fears and anxieties, guilt and excitement and a sense of loss (Falicov, 1998; Suarez-Orozco and Suarez-Orozco, 2002). The women in this study did experience challenges-as well as feelings of tension, stress and high anxiety throughout the actual move.

Step 1: Saying Goodbye. The trip to the airport including the time spent in the airport is characterized by an array of emotions including excitement and anticipation about the new country, the perceived opportunities for self and children, and the chance to escape earlier traumas such as maturational losses or adverse situations. These feelings are weighed against a variety of uncertainties: leaving loved ones (especially young children) behind, leaving friends, family, work, home, and a familiar environment. In many cases, the woman worries about what to expect upon her arrival, how to deal with her undocumented status, the possible complications of finding employment, how to find housing, supporting herself and her family at home, timely reunification with her children, the change in climate and a new environment. The immigrant woman's experience, already challenged by dealing with the stress of relocation, is further complicated by the difficulty of saying goodbye to loved ones, especially young children being left behind. Coping with the pain of saying goodbye to her children, and worrying about what to expect upon arrival, makes leaving extremely stressful for the immigrant woman. The woman deals with the stress in one of three ways: (1) *avoidance*: leaving the children at home to avoid the airport goodbyes–"There was no way I was going to take my son to the airport. I said goodbye to him at home"; (2) *denial*: pretending the trip is a vacation and the separation will be for a short period of time–"I just told my daughters that I was going to visit their cousin for a few months and would be back home before school started"; (3) *honest but controlled disclosure:* bringing loved ones to the airport and being honest with them about the indefinite period of separation. The third choice requires the woman to handle her own emotions as well as those of her children. In some cases, the woman suspends her feelings in an effort to make it easier on her children and/or herself: "I had mixed feelings. I was excited about leaving on the one hand, but I was also sad about leaving my children. But the whole time in the airport I just tried not to cry for my children's sake." Others are not always able to be stoic. "Both my children came to the airport with me. The little one cried a lot, but the older one ignored me. I wanted to be strong, but I broke down and cried." Another woman shared this experience: "At the airport, my little girl cried, and when I started walking to the plane she held on to my leg. She didn't want me to leave her." Women in this situation gain the strength needed to say goodbye by keeping in mind their goal of leaving for a better life. Family and friends who are part of the informal network often provide support at this point to help the woman remain focused on the long-term gains and to comfort the children.

Step 2: The Flight. The flight itself is another step in the relocation phase that is filled with ambiguities. The woman experiences exhilaration and anticipation of what is to come, but at the same time she is filled with fear and anxiety about the unknown. Some women fear the flight itself, which for many of them may be their first trip in a plane: "It was my first time on a plane, and I was a little scared." Since September 11, some women have an even greater fear of flying: "When I was coming on the plane, I tried hard not to think about 9/11. I kept praying I would get here safe and sound."

Step 3: Arrival and Immigration. For many women in the study, passing through Immigration generated a great deal of fear. Fear often is triggered by the simple act of completing the Immigration card, which asks the undocumented woman to indicate her place of residence upon arrival in the United States. Many women also become fearful during the long wait in the Immigration line and the often-intimidating interview with the Immigration officer. "I was drilled by the Immigration agent. I was shaking in my boots. This situation still affects me today, I still have nightmares of being sent back." Prior to migrating, some women had help preparing a "cover story" for the Immigration officer that helped them feel more confident. "I knew to keep my head down and be real polite. I practiced saying over and over. 'I am here to visit my grandmother.' " The women also experienced anxiety during the baggage inspection, and while searching for familiar faces in the waiting area to reassure them that they had in fact arrived and would not be sent back home.

Initial Adjustment

The adaptation to a new way of life presents a greater emotional challenge for women who migrate and leave their children than for those who do not. Adaptation to a new life, referred to as *acculturation* or *acculturation adjustment* has been defined as the degree of social, economic and psychological functioning a person has that enables him or her to adapt to a host culture (Kim and Nacissio, 1980). Acculturation is distinguished from assimilation, the "melting pot" ideology in which the values, customs and behaviors of the home country are integrated into the new country. Acculturation can be described also as a "culture change that results from continuous first-hand contact between two distinct cultural groups" (Berry, Minde, Kim, and Mok, 1987, p. 494). For Caribbean women, acculturation more accurately describes the process they experience as they adopt a bi-cultural lifestyle (Szapocznik & Kurtines, 1980).

The acculturation process for Caribbean immigrants is unique in some respects despite the fact that their countries of origin are geographically close in proximity to North America. Moving from a small tropical island to a large metropolis in North America presents unique challenges to the acculturation process, especially for women who leave their children behind. In the case of the Caribbean woman, acculturation can be experienced in several ways and to varying degrees; it can be viewed from a physical, psychological, economic, behavioral, educational, race and gender perspective. Most undocumented immigrants from the Caribbean come from the lower or middle socioeconomic classes, and they come to the United States to improve their lives economically and to provide their children with more financial and educational opportunities (Gopaul-McNicol, 1993). Because this may not be the case for every Caribbean woman who migrates to North America, acculturation varies depending on the woman's socioeconomic class and educational level. For example, a woman from a lower socioeconomic class will find that a job (even a domestic job) provides her with more money, which is a positive step because it helps her make a financial contribution to her family in the country of origin. On the other hand, a woman who is a professional (a teacher or a nurse) in her country of origin, and whose education, skills and years of experience are not accepted in the U.S., will have to adjust to working as a domestic or nurse's aide. The level of acculturative stress will be more severe for these women than for those from lower socioeconomic groups (Berry, 1997).

Race and class also can be significant to the acculturation process of the Caribbean immigrant. Although most immigrants know racism existed in the United States, they failed to see themselves as potential targets of racism. They had knowledge that racism existed for African Americans, but they thought that as foreigners they were exempt from it (Bashi-Bobb, 2001). Adjusting to overt racism and class discrimination can add to the stress of acculturation (Berry, 1997).

All of these factors, particularly the economic, educational, racial and class issues, influence the acculturation process of the Caribbean woman and contribute to the challenges she experiences as she adapts to a new society and a new way of life. In examining the acculturation process for the Caribbean woman, this study identifies three major steps women experience as part of this phase. These steps are not necessarily linear; they are progressive and can be cyclical at times during the acculturation stage.

Step 1: Relief and Hope. The first step of this stage occurs during the first few days and weeks in the new country. For many, it is described as the "honeymoon stage," a new and exciting time (Oberg, 1972, cited in Arredondo-Dowd, 1981). The woman displays a sense of relief that she has arrived safely after months, sometimes even years, of thinking and planning for the arrival day. One woman described the first few days: "I just wanted to walk, walk and walk around staring at the buildings and everything new. It was so different but it was exciting." Women describe this sense of hope as the sense that the dreams and positive opportunities for their children are now achievable. Even in the midst of strangers, women feel a sense of empowerment and excitement. "There was so much to do and see. I had never seen a train before or ridden on a bus like the ones in NYC. I just wanted to take it all in."

Step 2: Internal Struggling. For many women, the second step can begin after just a short time, as they begin to see the reality of their move. The woman's sense of guilt about being separated from her children, her feelings of loneliness, and the realization that her surroundings are different, become more noticeable and pronounced. The internal struggling becomes a daily occurrence. One woman described it: "I could see so many differences that were so positive. I was able to work. I was able to give things to my children. I was able to get an apartment. I was able to save money for when my children would come. And I found myself crying, crying and sometimes screaming at myself saying, `What have I done?' I would have nightmares about being separated from my kids. It was taking much longer to get my children than I ever expected."

It is in the internal struggling phase that a woman's resilience and desire for survival become paramount: "I had to keep going. I was determined that I would find a way to get my children here." One woman says, "This is the time I prayed more than I had ever prayed before. I prayed many times a day for my children, for the strength to keep going." Another woman states, "God is here to help me accomplish my goals. I am hoping I can accomplish what I want to in a certain amount of time." Women continue to seek internal strength and strength from other resources as they struggle with the challenges of incorporating the American culture into their day-to-day living. They also call upon a sense of faith and resilience as they work to achieve their dream and goal of being a legal immigrant and bringing their children to America. "God is here to help me with my goal. God is my strength."

Parenting from a distance or *transnational mothering*, as referred to by Pierrette Gondagneu-Sotelo and Ernestine Avilla (1997), further complicates the internal struggle for these women. As one woman puts it, "Either way it is hard. You can't win. The little ones listen when you speak to them by phone but it tears your heart to know you are not there with them to comb their hair and watch them grow up. As time goes by, sometimes I feel like they don't remember me. They call me mommy, but they are closer to their guardians than they are to me." When asked how she would describe herself as a mother, one woman responded by saying, "I am a mother who is lost because I don't have my children. We send each other pictures and we speak on the telephone but it is not the same." As these women explore their roles as mothers, they admit that they feel helpless: "I am not able to guide and protect my children, I am not able to raise them my way." Another mother states, "It frustrates me to give them advice on the telephone and know they are not taking it. My teenage daughter said to me, 'Where were you when I needed you?' I don't think I will ever forget that statement as long as I live." These women cope with long-distance parenting by providing their children with material goods (Salazar-Parrenas, 2001). They pack barrels filled with clothes and personal items that symbolize much more than the items in the barrel. The barrels are filled with love and, for these mothers, sending the barrels mean that they are good providers and good mothers. One mother explains, "I am able to buy my children all the necessities of life, these are things I am able to do now that I was not able to do before. I also send money to take care of them every month, it makes me feel good to do that for them." The continuing challenge for these immigrant women is balancing positive feelings about sending their children material goods and being a good provider with feelings of helplessness while parenting from a distance. During the internal struggling step, the role of the informal network in both the United States and the home country is an invaluable source of support for these women. "I sometimes go to my friends on weekends. I buy food that reminds me of home and we cook together. It makes me feel good." Another woman said, "When you work as a live-in, you have to work 24 hours a day. It is good to visit my aunt and my friends on the weekend." For immigrants today, contact with the country of origin is easier now than in the past because long-distance communication is readily available through telephone, fax and computers (Foner, 2001). For many, telephone contact is accessible and affordable. One woman states, "I called my friends at home. My friends would tell me, 'Your kids are fine. You can take care of your children better if you stay in America than if you come back. Stay and take care of yourself, so you can help your children.'" During the internal struggling step, the woman continues to struggle with conflicts and ambivalence about her choices. She may question her decision, especially as she faces the challenge of becoming legal and the greater challenge of bringing her children to this country. "I miss my family so much, sometimes I would call my husband and cry, but he always tell me to hold on a little longer, and remind me that I had given a lot of money to the lawyers to fix my papers and that things will work out." As the woman considers returning to her children and country of origin, she counteracts these feelings by (1) recalling life in her home country, (2) confirming her belief that life will be and can be better for her children in the U.S., and (3) thinking about the fear or embarrassment of returning and being seen as a failure.

Women report that they experience expected and unexpected situations that trigger the feelings of loss and ambivalence about their decision to move away from their children. When this happens, their sense of grief is enormous. One woman states, "When I see a child that physically resembles my daughter, for a split second I think it is my daughter. Then I become sad and realize I'm missing her a lot." These women experience grief continually, as they relive the initial feelings of disbelief, the moments of bargaining, the feelings of anger, and the sense of sadness and despair. During the acculturation process, women live and relive their losses and separations frequently: "Every time I sit to eat a meal, especially during the holidays, I wonder if they are eating."

Step 3: Resolve. The third step of the acculturation process involves resolve. It is at this time that the woman becomes able to function in her day-to-day life while managing the intensity of the previous step. She continues to experience conflict and internal struggles, but she has gained a level of understanding and coping: "I realized that bringing my children up is taking longer than I expected so I focus more on my work and buying things for my kids than on how much it hurts not to be with them." Working long hours seems to be a strategy these women use to cope. "I had three jobs sometimes when my children were home. I worked a day job, I had a night job three days a week and I worked weekends. I didn't want to think, so I just worked and worked." Others cope by becoming emotionally attached to the children they take care of. "I love the little boy I am taking care of–he is so loving. He is like my own child to me. I often find myself talking about him to people like he is my own child."

In this step, some women reach out to others in their home country and become that informal network for those who might want to come to America. When women were asked the question, "Knowing what you know now, what might you say to a woman who is thinking of coming to America and has to leave her kids," several commented on the difficulties involved. One woman's response was, " I would tell them to come, but I would also say that it is very painful and stressful leaving your children. It is a pain that you never forget. The pain and the experience are unbearable. But in the long run, there are gains because they can live here better than at home." One woman who reflects on her experience states, "If I had known how long and hard it would have been to get my children here and the pain of being separated from them, I would never have left my country." Some said they had trouble forgiving themselves: "I have never forgiven myself for what I did to my children." Another woman responded, "It is not easy leaving your children. However, if you are as determined as I was, you can do it. I am 'home' now here in America and my children are here with me."

CONCLUSIONS AND RECOMMENDATIONS

The Caribbean immigrant women's study is a qualitative study with a structured instrument for data collection. Integral milestones have been identified to provide a more comprehensive framework for exploring the decision-making process for women. For Caribbean women who may be considering leaving their home country, this study identifies significant steps and resources to access that are integral to the migratory process. For Caribbean women who have left their children behind, this study can be used to identify and emphasize the internal and external resources that were used at different steps in the decision-making process. It is these resources that can strengthen the woman's sense of self, support and enhance the parent-child relationship during the separation, and provide support with the grieving process.

Both the study and the model suggest that the decision-making process is a painful and traumatic experience that has many implications for children and mothers alike. Families from developing countries search for a better life, and the first world's demand for service workers creates the motivation for women (and by extension, mothers) to migrate, resulting in mothers separating from their children for long and indefinite periods of time.

The authors do not mean to suggest that the stressors of the separation caused by migration in and of itself mean that transnational families are pathological. However, it is important to recognize that the stressors caused by the separation and the accompanying grieving process may impact the adjustment stage. It would be beneficial for practitioners to become familiar with the separation and loss issues inherent in the migratory process for transnational families.

Additional studies in the future are needed to support women who migrate and, in particular, women who are left parenting their children from a distance. Research on the child's perspective would be helpful in understanding how the child experiences the mother's migratory process and the effects of parenting from a distance. It would also be useful to identify specific strategies to correspond with the various steps women experience in the decision-making process, to assist with the strengthening and maintenance of the parent/child relationship before, during and after migration. Also, it is critical for the field to develop strategies for transnational families to help parents cope with separation and loss, and help their child(ren) with their own experience with separation and loss due to immigration. These strategies need to be utilized to maintain and ultimately strengthen the mother/child attachment both during the period of separation, as well as through the process of reunification.

The findings gathered in this study are not as conclusive as a study of a representative sample of immigrant women from the Caribbean who have left their children behind: Because of the small sample, the findings cannot be generalized to the overall immigrant population. But the study does give a snapshot of the decision-making process for women in this region of the world who are or have had to separate from their children.

REFERENCES

Arredondo-Dowd, P. M. (1981). "Personal Loss and Grief as a Result of Immigration." *The Personnel and Guidance Journal*, 59(6), 376-378.

Basch, L. (2001). "Transnational Social Relations and the Politics of National Identity: An Eastern Caribbean Case Study." In Nancy Foner (Ed.). *Islands in the City: West Indian Migration to New York*. Berkeley: University of California Press.

Bashi-Bobb, V. (2001). "Neither Ignorance nor Bliss: Race, Racism and the West Indian Immigrant Experience." In Cordero-Guzman, Smith, & Grosfoguel (Eds.). *Migration, Transnationalization, and Race in a Changing New York*. Philadelphia: Temple University Press.

Berry, J. W., Kim, U., Minde, T., & Mok, D. (1987). "Comparative Studies of Acculturative Stress." *International Migration Review*, 21, 491-511.

Berry, J. W. (1997). "Immigration, Acculturation and Adaptation." *Applied Psychology*, 46: 5-68.

Bowlby, J. (1961). "Process of Mourning." *International Journal of Psycho-Analytic*. 42:317-40.

Chang, G. (2000). *Disposable Domestics: Immigrant Women Workers in the Global Economy*. Cambridge: South End Press.

Donato, K. (1992). "Understanding U.S. Immigration: Why Some Countries Send Women and Others Send Men." In Donna Gabaccia (Ed.). *Seeking Common Ground: Multidisciplinary Studies of Immigrant Women in the United States*. Westport, CT: Praeger.

Espin, O. M. (1987). "Psychological Impact of Migration on Latinas: Implications for Psychotherapeutic Practice." *Psychology of Women Quarterly*, 11, 480-503.

Falicov, C. J. (1998). *Latino Families in Therapy: A Guide to Multicultural Practice*. New York: Guilford Press.

Foner, N. (1985). "Race and Color: Jamaican Migrants in London and New York City." *International Migration Review*, 19 (4): 708-27.

Foner, N., Rumbaut, R. G., & Gold, S. J. (2000). *Immigration Research for a New Century: Multidisciplinary Perspectives*. New York: Russell Sage Foundation.

Foner, N. (2001). *Islands in the City: West Indian Migration to New York*. Los Angeles: University of California Press.

Foner, N. (2001). "Transnationalism Then and Now: New York Immigrants Today and at the Turn of the Twentieth Century." In Cordero-Guzman, Smith, & Grosfoguel (eds). *Migration, Transnationalization, and Race in a Changing New York*. Philadelphia: Temple University Press.

Foner, N. (2001). "Introduction: New Immigrants in New York." In Foner (Ed). *New Immigrants in New York*. New York: Columbia University Press.

Gopaul-McNicol, S. (1993). *Working with West Indian Families.* New York: The Guilford Press.

Hondagneu-Sotelo, P. (1992). "Overcoming Patriarchal Constraints: The Reconstruction of Gender Relations Among Mexican Immigrant Women and Men." *Gender and Society,* 6, 393-415.

Hondagneu-Sotelo, P. & Avilla, E. (1997). "I am Here, But I'm There: The Meaning of Latina Transnational Motherhood." *Gender and Society,* 11: 548-71.

Houston, M., Kramer, R., & Mackin-Barrett, J. (1984). "Female Predominance of Immigration to the United States Since 1930: A First Look." *International Migration Review,* 18: 908-63.

Kasinitz, P. & Vickerman, M. (2001). "Ethnic Niches and Racial Traps: Jamaicans in the New York Regional Economy." In Cordero-Guzman, Smith, & Grosfoguel (eds). *Migration, Transnationalization, and Race in a Changing New York.* Philadelphia: Temple University Press.

Keith, V. M. & Herring, C. (1991). "Skin Tone and Stratification in the Black Community." *American Journal of Sociology,* 97 (3) 760-79.

Kim, Y. Y. & Nicassio, P. M. (1980). *Research Project on Indochinese Refugees in the State of Illinois: Survey of Indochinese: Methods and Procedures, II.* Chicago: Aldine.

Kübler-Ross (1969). *On Death and Dying.* New York: Collier Books.

New York City Department of City Planning (1996). "The Newest New Yorkers: An Analysis of Immigration to NYC in the Early 1990's."

Portes, A. & Stepick, A. (1993). *City on the Edge: The Transformation of Miami.* Berkeley: University of California Press.

Ricketts, E. (1987). "U.S. Investment and Immigration from the Caribbean." *Social Problems,* 34 (4): 374-87.

Salazar-Parrenas, R. (2001). "Mothering From a Distance: Emotions, Gender, and Intergenerational Relations in Filipino Transnational Families." *Feminist Studies,* 27 (2) 361-390.

Salvo, J. & Ortiz, R. (1992). *The Newest New Yorkers: An analysis of Immigration into New York City During the 1980s.* New York City: New York City Department of City Planning.

Sassen, S. (1988). "America's Immigration 'Problem.'" *World Policy Journal,* 6: 811-32.

Sassen, S. (1988). *The Mobility of Labor and Capital: A Study in International Investment and Labor Flow.* Cambridge: Cambridge University Press.

Soto, I. M. (1987). "West Indian Child Fostering: Its Role in Migrant Exchanges." In Constance R. Sutton & Elsa M. Chaney (Eds.). *Caribbean Life in New York City: Sociocultural Dimensions.* New York: Center for Migration Studies.

Suarez-Orozco, C. & Suarez-Orozco, M. (2002). *Children of Immigration: The Developing Child Series.* Cambridge, MA: Harvard University Press.

Szapoeznik, J. & Kurtines, W. (1980). "Acculturation, Biculturalism and Adjustment Among Cuban Americans." In A. Padilla (ed.). *Acculturation: Theory Models and Some New Findings* (139-159). Boulder, CO: Westview Press.

Waldinger, R. (1996). *Still the Promise City: African Americans and New Immigrants in Post Industrial New York.* Cambridge: Harvard University Press.

Watkins-Owens, I. (2001). "Early-Twentieth-Century Caribbean Women: Migration and Social Networks in New York City." In Nancy, Foner, (Ed.). *Islands in the City: West Indian Migration to New York.* Los Angeles: University of California Press.

Zhou, M. (1992). *Chinatown: The Socioeconomic Potential of an Urban Enclave.* Philadelphia: Temple University Press.

Developing a Model Intervention
to Prevent Abuse
in Relationships Among Caribbean
and Caribbean-American Youth
by Partnering with Schools

Kristine A. Herman

SUMMARY. This paper proposes a model intervention to prevent relationship abuse among Caribbean and Caribbean-American adolescents. Specifically, the model partners with a high school with a strong Caribbean student population and incorporates education, prevention and intervention, as the three core components. This paper highlights the importance of working with young people in a school setting, working with young people before they have fully tackled the developmental task of defining norms of and values in relationships, utilizing culturally competent staff and specialized programming, and emphasizing the need for early intervention in the instances of adolescent relationship violence before its evolution into adult domestic violence. The model proposed serves as an outline for further development of culturally-specific and compe-

Kristine A. Herman, Esq., MSW, is Coordinator of Special Projects, Domestic Violence Programs at the Center for Court Innovation, 520 Eighth Avenue, 18th Floor, New York, NY 10018.

[Haworth co-indexing entry note]: "Developing a Model Intervention to Prevent Abuse in Relationships Among Caribbean and Caribbean-American Youth by Partnering with Schools." Herman, Kristine A. Co-published simultaneously in *Journal of Immigrant & Refugee Services* (The Haworth Social Work Practice Press, an imprint of The Haworth Press, Inc.) Vol. 2, No. 3/4, 2004, pp. 103-116; and: *The Health and Well-Being of Caribbean Immigrants in the United States* (ed: Annette M. Mahoney) The Haworth Social Work Practice Press, an imprint of The Haworth Press, Inc., 2004, pp. 103-116. Single or multiple copies of this article are available for a fee from The Haworth Document Delivery Service [1-800-HAWORTH, 9:00 a.m. - 5:00 p.m. (EST). E-mail address: docdelivery@haworthpress.com].

tent interventions to prevent and address relationship violence among adolescents. *[Article copies available for a fee from The Haworth Document Delivery Service: 1-800-HAWORTH. E-mail address: <docdelivery@haworth press.com> Website: <http://www.HaworthPress.com> © 2004 by The Haworth Press, Inc. All rights reserved.]*

KEYWORDS. Caribbean (persons born in an English-speaking Caribbean island and who have immigrated to the United States), Caribbean-American (second generation children of Caribbean immigrants), adolescents (young people between the ages of 14-19 years)

In the United States, young women between the ages of 16-24 in dating relationships experience the highest rate of domestic violence and sexual assault. In a study of five hundred New York City adolescents, between 17% and 23% reported being intimidated, threatened, hit or slapped by their partner, and an additional 25% reported verbal abuse such as humiliation, insults and embarrassment. Another study of more than six hundred high school students reported that almost one third of those surveyed interpreted violent acts as acts of love. The average prevalence rate of nonsexual dating violence, as summarized by the National Center for Injury Prevention and Control, is 22% among high school students (Sugarman & Hotaling, 1989). A study of eighth and ninth grade students showed that 25% of them had been victims of nonsexual dating violence and 8% had been victims of sexual dating violence (Foshee et al., 1996). While many studies explore estimates broken down by race on the prevalence of relationship violence in adolescents, there is a notable absence of statistics on Caribbean and Caribbean-American adolescents who are victims of relationship violence.

However, the overall prevalence of relationship violence among adolescents indicates a substantial need to provide specialized programming aimed at reducing dating violence against young women and girls. This paper proposes a model program that aims to prevent adult domestic violence by interrupting the cycle of violence at its earliest stage. Specifically, this model intervention is designed to address the unique needs and issues of Caribbean and Caribbean-American adolescents living in the United States who may be victims, perpetrators or at risk for victimization or perpetration of relationship violence.

ABUSE IN ADOLESCENT RELATIONSHIPS

Abuse in adolescent relationships, frequently referred to as teen dating violence, is unique from adult domestic violence in several important ways. During the adolescent and young adulthood process of moving from dependence to independence, adolescents establish complex peer relationships and have their first experiences with intimate relationships. It is through this process that adolescents develop beliefs and attitudes about who they are and what kind of person they want to be.

Recent literature on theories of psychological development report differences in the way adolescent girls develop when compared to adolescent boys. For adolescent girls, development of a sense of self and morality "takes place through an understanding of the psychological logic of relationships" (Gilligan, 1983). For boys and men, separation and individuation may be critically tied to gender identity, but for girls and women issues of femininity and a feminine identity are not necessarily dependent on the achievement of such separation and individuation. Gilligan mentions Jean Baker Miller's observations that in the course of female development, young women and girls paradoxically keep large parts of themselves out of relationship in their attempt to make and maintain relationships (Gilligan, 1983).

It is in this context that teens may become involved in relationships that are unequal or abusive. Teen dating violence is distinguished from adult domestic violence by adolescents' inexperience in intimate relationships, making it difficult for them to recognize signs of abuse and more likely to romanticize abusive behavior. Adolescents may enter relationships with inappropriate, unhealthy or abusive expectations based on cultural and gender-role stereotypes. As teens become socialized into gender roles, these roles are influenced by culturally-specific ideas of gender and can put pressure on adolescents to conform to these expectations and accept the limitations such cultured gender stereotypes offer.

CULTURAL FACTORS

Issues of youth development and relationship violence are further complicated by cultural factors for Caribbean and second generation Caribbean youth. Specifically, work with Caribbean youths and families around issues of relationship violence must include an understanding and awareness of the cultural factors that impact young people, such as: immigration issues and the second generation issues of Caribbean immigrants, and Caribbean families' and community thinking around relationships, violence, gender roles and sexuality.

Caribbean Americans from English-speaking republics frequently come to the United States with professional and business backgrounds and a fluency in English. However, these immigrant advantages are summarily lost once they have arrived to find that the context in which they are quickly placed is that of native-born Black Americans who are subject to discrimination and racial prejudice (Portes & Zhou, 1999). For this reason, Caribbean immigrants may resist acculturation in the United States, resist identifying racially with African Americans and strive to retain their Caribbean cultural identity (Kassinitz, 1993). For Caribbean immigrants the issues of race and ethnicity have different meanings and such divisions typically are not directly linked to status in their countries of origin. Once in the United States, however, there is a noticeable downward status shift as Caribbean immigrants become identified as part of Black America. Whereas once they were part of a majority where race was not superbly indicative of social mobility (though arguably class and color distinctions were), now they find themselves part of an oppressed minority (Kassinitz, 1992). It is in this context that Caribbean immigrants cling to their cultural identity, resist assimilation and attempt to hold at bay their racial identity (Waters & Eschback, 1999).

For adolescent children of Caribbean immigrants, the conflict between a cultural identity and a racial one is even stronger. While there may be pressure from parents and their community to retain-cultural values and behavior, there is also a push to realize the American Dream and to adopt values of American society and American youth culture.

Culturally enforced gender roles and strict expectations of behavior around issues such as dating and interpersonal relationships can lead to complex responses among adolescents when the cultural messages of American youth conflict with the strict restraints often put on behavior (particularly the behavior of young girls) by Caribbean families and community. Sociologists have noted that these culturally-determined gender-specific pressures can often push young women towards a more Americanized lifestyle, including everything from wanting more freedom to date and stay out late, to promiscuity, to wanting greater gender equality (Waters, 1999). The Caribbean and Caribbean-American adolescent embarking on the developmental tasks of individuation and differentiation can run head-on into the beliefs and values of their parents. The individual rights afforded youth in the United States and the strong social messages that view young people as independent actors may run against the Caribbean traditions and messages. These adolescents can suffer intense family conflict based on intra-family cultural differences and competing norms.

It is in is this context that the stark difference between culturally defined gender roles, what is culturally defined as "acceptable" behavior for girls, runs head-on into American versions of individualization, independence and (frequently to the displeasure of immigrant parents) a new concept of female sexuality for adolescent girls. These culture conflicts can lead to difficult tensions within Caribbean families trying to navigate the space between first and second-generation immigrants. The cultural differences in gender roles, identity and family attitudes frequently clash with the messages young people receive at school, from their peers and in American society in general.

The tension experienced by Caribbean and Caribbean-American adolescents to be more "American" and to move further away from their culture of origin can raise a series of concerns that include: a lack of healthy teen relationship models, a lack of parental and community support for interpersonal and dating relationship behaviors, and a lack of education, resources, or guidance as they explore the issues of intimacy, relationships, and gender equality within relationships. Caribbean and Caribbean-American adolescents frequently walk a tightrope between the cultural norms that are rooted in the Caribbean and the values and norms of a new American society, one which neither the youth nor the young person's families may be ready and equipped to fully adapt to. Adolescents in Caribbean immigrant families are subject to multiple and difficult conflicting cultural and social demands (Portes & Zhou, 1999). This cultural tightrope walk or social straddling of sorts can result in a barrage of mixed messages and competing signals about what is a healthy relationship and what constitutes abuse in a relationship. Yet there is no other population in domestic violence literature that has received less attention than that of Caribbean adolescents, their relationships and relationship violence among Caribbean and Caribbean-American youth.

A SCHOOL-BASED MODEL

School is the place where young people spend most of their day and form most of their social relationships; it is the most important institution and setting in the lives of adolescents because it is where they test most of their developing relational skills, communication skills, values, beliefs, and sense of identity. Additionally, school is where Caribbean and Caribbean-American youths come face-to-face with prevalent cultural norms of Black America and choose what to adopt, and whether to assimilate or retain cultural norms of their country of origin. It is in school that youths form most of their peer relationships, which are frequently defined through race-based groupings. Consequently, school is the key place to implement a model program to prevent adult domestic violence, reduce teen relationship violence, and educate students, teachers and parents about relationship violence in the Caribbean and Caribbean-American community.

Young people who experience relationship violence learn that a certain level of violence is normal, and therefore develop a framework for selecting partners and evaluating relationships based on that idea. Experiencing relationship violence as an adolescent can lead to the development of beliefs that violence, possessiveness, jealousy, and controlling behavior are an expected and inevitable part of a romantic involvement. The need for prevention and intervention efforts early in the development of young people is highlighted by studies showing a connection between teen dating violence and adult domestic violence, with young people involved in violent dating relationships expressing greater acceptance of violence in marriages (Gamache, 1990).

A model school-based program to prevent abuse in relationships among Caribbean and Caribbean-American youth utilizes multiple practice methods and includes three-part programming: *prevention, education* and *intervention*. *Prevention* is an integral part of a relationship violence program because it proactively promotes the development of healthy relationships, changes the culture of the school, and raises awareness about a serious underreported social issue. *Education* is critical to help professionals identify and understand the prevalence of dating violence, make appropriate referrals, and respond appropriately to dating violence situations in the school. This allows school personnel to be better equipped to address dating violence, and also assists in creating a climate where the uniform message is that violence against a dating partner will not be tolerated. *Intervention* is critical to address issues that manifest early in a young person's life before they escalate to adult domestic violence, substance abuse, dropout, suicide or involvement in the criminal justice system.

A model school-based relationship violence program empowers young women and girls, raises awareness at the school, parent and community level, provides educational groups for adolescents at risk for perpetrating relationship violence, and provides much-needed support and services to adolescent victims of relationship violence. Such a school-based program could not address the difficult issue of relationship violence in a vacuum stripped of all cultural differences, biases and beliefs. Thus it is imperative that any program seeking to undertake the issue of relationship violence among teens be culturally-competent and includes culturally-relevant issues in the ongoing dialogue. Support services should demonstrate a competency in the realities of the Caribbean and Caribbean-American adolescents and an ability to offer healthy guidance during this time of identity formation. A model program must be culturally sensitive to issues of family conflict, varying beliefs in corporal punishment, differences in expressions and body language, and issues of gender and class. Without an evidenced understanding of social and cultural differences, no program would succeed in reaching the young people who straddle the fence between the Caribbean community and American society.

HOW IT WORKS

A model intervention to prevent abuse in relationships among Caribbean and Caribbean-American youth utilizes all elements of direct social work practice: relationship, assessment, communication, self-awareness/use of self, and intervention. This model is designed to address the needs of individuals and groups within the context of community and culture. While the bulk of the model revolves around group work, other practice methods are used in the intervention strategies, such as direct clinical practice with individual victims and perpetrators of relationship violence when necessary, interviewing and assessment for students referred to the groups, and community practice in the outreach efforts to raise parent and community awareness and promote community change on the issue of relationship violence.

Student Awareness. All students at the high school should be eligible for a classroom-based multi-session curriculum. Teachers should consent to allow curriculum facilitators access to the classroom to provide school-wide education on relationship violence one classroom at a time. The curriculum is a one-to-three session classroom-based training on the definition of relationship and dating violence, the signs of relationship violence, legal and social community resources for victims of relationship violence, the law around relationship violence, and information on the cycle of violence. Activities can include an exercise asking young people to reflect and record the different spheres of their lives in which they receive information about relationships and gender roles, and then a discussion can be lead to what those messages are and how they conflict with each other, where gaps might be, and highlighting the different messages women and girls receive compared to their male counterparts. Explorations into language and the use of language to oppress and perpetuate sexism and racism can be of use to stimulate discussions about gender and male privilege.

A powerful component of an in-school relationship violence prevention campaign includes student-facilitated discussions and activities. One such example occurred during a student-run after-school discussion group on relationship violence, where two trained female students outlined the cycle of violence and gave other students vignettes and asked them to decide if they thought that met their definition of abusive behavior. When the students in the room were split, as they frequently were, students explained their perspective on why certain behaviors were and were not violent. One young man in the group expressed his view that Caribbean men have a duty and a right to physically correct women, even if that means pushing, hitting or strangling her to get a point across. This young man's comment was met by several young women's views that his notion of his rights as a Caribbean male were outdated and that as young women they would not accept such behavior from a boyfriend. In another coeducational group held in the school's counseling center during students' lunch hour, students expressed varying opinions on possessiveness, jealousy and controlling behaviors. In this context students were given a forum to challenge each other's beliefs and set new norms for developing healthy relationships.

Pamphlets, designed to educate young people about dating violence and address the unique safety issues for teen victims of relationship violence, outline the risk factors and indicators of relationship violence, and provide information on resources for teenage victims of relationship violence, are to be available at the school. Pamphlets are distributed to students at the end of each classroom-based curriculum on relationship violence and are made available for students to pick up throughout the high school in classrooms, offices and public spaces.

School Staff Awareness. All teachers and school personnel should be eligible and strongly encouraged by the high school principal to participate in a school awareness workshop on dating violence to learn the warning signs, understand the cycle of violence and the prevalence and scope of the problem, and to get tools and supports for addressing issues of relationship violence in the school setting. Teachers are trained in the Department of Education sexual harassment policy, and this policy serves as the foundation for enforcement in cases of gender-based violence and abuse. Additionally, in the school staff awareness trainings, teachers learn to identify relationship abuse in the school and other high-risk behaviors of young people. Teachers are to report incidents of suspected relationship violence to the Principal or Vice Principal/Head of Guidance at the school for disciplinary action. The goal of this professional development training is to provide teachers, guidance counselors, mediators, secretaries, janitorial staff and any staff member who may witness student interactions, with the skills and resources they need to intervene, respond and refer to cases of dating violence. The training should be led by two co-facilitators who are experts in the area of relationship violence and who reflect the cultural backgrounds of the students.

The principal, teachers and staff frequently set the tone and culture of the school in their policies and practice when responding to incidents of relationship violence against students. One school in New York City recently had an incident where a number of students sexually assaulted a female student in school, and the response to the incident by the school administration neglected any services or special programming for the young men involved in the assault, neglected to involve the on-site police officer, as schools in New York are ranked according to levels of dangerousness and criminal arrests on campus, and neglected to provide services to the victim of the assault. This school is an example of the lack of training and innovative strategies available to teachers and administrators to properly address incidents of relationship and sexual violence in school. Similarly, in this incident the young woman's parents did not want to damage the future of the young men involved in the assault, thus no charges were filed and the in-school disciplinary action taken was minimal and not specially targeted to address the offense in question.

Parent/Community Awareness. All parents of high school students should be notified by mail of a community forum on dating violence. The parent/community forum should be held at school in the evening, and should run approximately two hours in length. The forum should be facilitated by program staff, and co-hosted by students at the high school. The forum serves as an opportunity for students, program staff, teachers, and school personnel to raise awareness about the problem of relationship violence in the school and in the community. Additionally, outreach efforts to specific parents should be made in instances where young people involved in the intervention groups consent.

Reliance on new lines of cultural transmission should be utilized, so that as students' perspectives around the issue of relationship violence change so, too, may the parents. At the school level, education as cultural transmission is realized in the interaction of generations, but fundamental in this interaction process is the reciprocity of cultural transmission: both actors in the interaction process, educators, adults as well as children, contribute to cultural transmission. Although many educators, parents as well as teachers, are trying to transmit very explicitly and intentionally selected parts of their culture and differing cultural messages to their children and pupils, their behavior is not only directed by their own intentions, but also by the managing behavior of young people. Therefore, reciprocity may result in a new form of cultural socialization for the entire family through direct family socialization and indirect influence of social relationships at large.

Intervention. Mandatory and voluntary school-based intervention groups are held for ten-week cycles, with rolling admission so students can be referred to the group at any time during the school year and he/she will still complete the full ten sessions. Groups are gender-specific and cover topics such as goal-setting, defining abuse, language, gender stereotypes, positive vs. negative self-talk, quick fixes, relationship/negative consequence history, personal relevance, cultural messages and socialization, homophobia and a weekly check-in. The groups target students who are perpetrators, of dating violence or at high risk for becoming perpetrators, and students who are victims of dating violence.

Once an incident has come to the attention of the Principal or the Vice Principal/Head of Guidance, if the incident allows for administrative discretion, the Principal or Vice Principal mandates participation in an Early Intervention Group as a condition of remaining in school. Thus, an Early Intervention Group is used as an alternative to suspension, similar to many schools' already existing policy of in-school afternoon suspension (wherein students stay after school several afternoons a week as an alternative to suspension). Students mandated to the group are referred by the Principal or Vice Principal's completion of a referral form.

Each group should be held once per week and have a maximum enrollment of ten participants. Groups may be held after school or during lunch, so as not to disrupt the students' class schedules. Students for the gender-specific early intervention groups should be identified through a variety of possible referral sources: youth court, school principal, guidance counselors, teachers, parents, Mediation Center, probation, police, and court.

The group uses a direct clinical social work practice method, using group work strategies, and the intervention is gender-based, with the young men's early intervention group consisting of mandatory referrals from several referral sources, and the young women's group being voluntary and referral-based. Any young men identified as victims of relationship violence are not to be referred to the mandatory early intervention group for young men (as it will be designed to focus on the unique needs of adolescent perpetrators of relationship violence), but instead are to be seen on an individual basis by a Group Facilitator until an outside referral could be made to an appropriate social service agency. Similarly, if a young woman is identified as the abuser in a relationship, she may be screened out of the young women's early intervention group and could be seen individually by a Group Facilitator until an appropriate referral could be made.

Young Men's Early Intervention Group. For young men mandated to the Early Intervention Group, prior to the intake interview, a Group Facilitator should gather as much information from the referral source and other professionals, teachers, staff, etc. Information gathered should include: a written referral form completed by referring agency or staff member, a follow-up conversation with the referral source, a detailed history of the disciplinary action taken by the school, agency or court, investigating whether this person has access to weapons and is involved in a gang, getting a history of school or program attendance, checking to see if the young person is involved in a special needs program or is learning disabled, getting a mental health history if possible and a list of any medications the young person may have been prescribed, and compiling information about substance use and any court involvement the young person may currently have. The Early Intervention Group Facilitator should administer an intake questionnaire (similar to an assessment instrument) designed to determine eligibility and appropriateness for the Early Intervention Group, and any possible barriers to participation in the Group; the intake interview serves to establish a trusting working relationship while allowing the young person to explore why they have been referred to the group and how the group can help them.

A Group Facilitator should consider the following indicators of youth at risk for dating violence:

- uses size to intimidate females and is intimidating to others
- has negative verbal outbursts
- uses inappropriate sexual language towards females and/or is degrading towards females
- has problems relating to female students or adult women and/or difficulty interacting with females
- has had incidents of abusing a mother or female figure in the household
- loses temper quickly
- has attitude that women or girls are at the source of problems for men or boys
- engages in sexual harassment and/or inappropriate physical contact
- witnessed domestic violence in the home
- engages in physical intimidation against a female guardian or female teacher
- has strict ideas of gender roles

Once an intake has been completed, the young person is required to sign the Group Contract in order to be admitted to the group. Through the contract used in the group, the student commits to nonviolence and agrees to talk openly in the group. The Group Contract also allows the Group Facilitator to give information about the young person's progress to others as agreed to and named by the young person and facilitator (such as parents, guardians, probation officer, guidance counselor, and other).

A perfect candidate for the Young Men's Early Intervention Group was a young man named Alex. Alex was a sixteen-year-old boy who had problems in school with female teachers and was arrested for physically assaulting his mother. Alex was referred for an intake and through the interview process it was discovered that Alex's dad had been arrested for domestic violence against Alex's mom earlier in the year, that the dad was currently out of the house with an order of protection against him, and that Alex had grown up in a home with domestic violence. Alex was aware of the violence he had witnessed at home, was angry with his father for how he treated his mother, and was clear that he did not want to become like his father, yet he was involved in the criminal justice system for domestic violence. Alex's mother did not understand that the violence Alex was perpetrating now against her and female teachers could one day extend to intimate relationships and adult domestic violence, and that this was a learned behavior that wasn't being addressed. Alex's referral to a young men's early intervention group was critical in attempting to halt the cycle of violence that Alex had learned at home.

Young Women's Early Intervention Group. For young women referred to the Early Intervention Group, a facilitator gathers as much information from the referral source and other professionals, teachers, staff, etc., as possible. Information gathered should include: a written referral form completed by referring agency or staff member, a follow-up conversation with the referral source, reason for the referral, checking to see if the young person is involved in a special needs program or is learning disabled, getting a mental health history if possible and a list of any medications the young person may have been prescribed, and compiling information about substance use and any court involvement the young person may currently have.

Teachers, staff, counselors and other school personnel should be trained in the school staff awareness training to identify indicators and risk factors for young women at risk for being a victim of relationship abuse. Warning signs of youth at risk for being a victim of dating violence include:

- physical marks or bruises
- changes in dress or makeup
- failing grades or withdrawal from school activities
- difficulty making decisions
- depression, mood changes and/or alcohol or drug use
- flat affect when reporting incidents of violence in a relationship
- willingness to stay in a relationship at all costs
- being totally focused on their partner's needs and wants
- minimization of violence
- self-blame and accentuating her role in perpetuating the abuse
- violent outbursts and perpetration of violence themselves

The Group Facilitator for the Young Women's Early Intervention Group should be a female who is knowledgeable in and representative of the cultural backgrounds of the students. The intake interview serves to establish a trusting working relationship and allows the young person to explore why they have been referred to the group and how the group can help them. The group should cover issues such as safety planning, identifying patterns of abusive behavior, and lessons on healthy relationships and respect, and should be aimed at empowering young women and educating them about community resources for victims of relationship violence.

In order to facilitate referrals to the mandatory young men's group and the voluntary young women's group, outreach should be conducted by Group Facilitators, prevention counselors, guidance counselors, probation officers, mediators and other school personnel. Fliers advertising groups should be posted in the school, as should educational posters aimed at continuing to raise awareness of relationship violence. Additionally, the school principal should be encouraged to use the young men's group as an alternative disciplinary tool when appropriate.

CONCLUSION AND RECOMMENDATIONS

A model program to prevent abuse in relationships among adolescents is a crucial next step in developing innovative and effective strategies to prevent domestic violence in the Caribbean and Caribbean-American community. Further analysis is necessary to explore policy and educational implications of cultural transmission techniques on a range of issues, from immigration and assimilation, to gender role attitudes and beliefs and the effectiveness of the school-based intervention and prevention model with Caribbean and Caribbean-American young people and their families. The extent to which young immigrant adolescents and children of immigrants are able to reciprocally transmit and influence their families' beliefs and values around relationship violence has not yet been fully explored.

A school-based program targeted to Caribbean and Caribbean-American adolescents, who are walking the tightrope between conflicting cultural beliefs, and who are actively engaged in the developmental tasks of individualization, formation of identity, gender roles, understanding and testing cultural and social norms, relationship-building and formulating values and beliefs in relationships, is critical to preventing abuse in relationships among Caribbean and Caribbean-American youth and is crucial to the larger struggle of preventing and eradicating adult domestic violence in American society as a whole.

REFERENCES

Foshee, V.A., Linder, G.F., Bauman, K.E., Langwick, S.A., Arriaga, X.B., Heath, J.L., McMahon, P.M., & Bangdiwala, S. (1996). "The Safe Dates Project: Theoretical Basis, Evaluation Design, and Selected Baseline Finding." Youth Violence Prevention: Description and Baseline Data from 13 Evaluation Projects (K. Powell & D.

Hawkins, Eds.). *American Journal of Preventative Medicine*, Supplement, Vol. 12, No. 5, 39-47.

Gilligan, C. (1983). *In a Different Voice: Psychological Theory and Women's Development*. Cambridge, MA: Harvard University Press.

Kassinitz, P. (1993). *Caribbean New York: Black Immigrants: The Politics of Race. New York: Cornell University Press.*

Portes, A. & Zhou, M. (1999). The New Second Generation: Segmented Assimilation and its variants. In N. Yetman (Ed.), *Majority and Minority: The Dynamics of Race and Ethnicity in American Life*. Massachusetts: Alyn and Bacon.

Sugarman, D.B. and Hotaling, G.T. (1989). "Dating Violence: Prevalence, Context, and Risk Markers." In M.A. Pirog-Good, & J.E. Stets, (Eds.), *Violence in Dating Relationships*. New York: Praeger, 3-32.

Waters, M. (1999). *Black Identities: West Indian Immigrant Dreams and American Realities*. Russell Sage Foundation, Harvard University Press.

Waters, K. & Eschbach, K. (1999). Immigration and Ethnic and Racial Inequality in the United States. In N. Yetman (Ed.), *Majority and Minority: The Dynamics of Race and Ethnicity in American Life*. Massachusetts: Allyn and Bacon.

Protecting Victims
of Domestic Violence
in Caribbean Communities

Mary Spooner

SUMMARY. A decade after the courts in many English-speaking Caribbean jurisdictions were granted the power to issue restraining orders to victims of domestic violence, battered women have not experienced the full benefits of such policy. Using the experiences of battered women in the English-speaking Caribbean state of Barbados, this study argues that there are significant challenges for victims, caused by cultural, social and economic factors that have not been appropriately addressed by domestic violence legislation. Marginalized by the court and legal system in the English-speaking Caribbean, many battered women seek out alternatives to the legal system for coping with domestic violence. Therefore when they migrate to countries like the United States where more accommodations are made for victims of domestic violence, they

Mary Spooner, PhD, is Program Evaluation Director, Holy Cross Children's Services, 8759 Clinton-Macon Road, Clinton, MI 49236.

The author would like to acknowledge the tremendous support of Dr. Randy Albelda and Dr. Paula Aymer through the numerous revisions of her ongoing work. She is extremely grateful to the women who took part in this study, the key informants, law enforcement and court personnel who shared their knowledge and in other ways facilitated her research.

[Haworth co-indexing entry note]: "Protecting Victims of Domestic Violence in Caribbean Communities." Spooner, Mary. Co-published simultaneously in *Journal of Immigrant & Refugee Services* (The Haworth Social Work Practice Press, an imprint of The Haworth Press, Inc.) Vol. 2, No. 3/4, 2004, pp. 117-134; and: *The Health and Well-Being of Caribbean Immigrants in the United States* (ed: Annette M. Mahoney) The Haworth Social Work Practice Press, an imprint of The Haworth Press, Inc., 2004, pp. 117-134. Single or multiple copies of this article are available for a fee from The Haworth Document Delivery Service [1-800-HAWORTH, 9:00 a.m. - 5:00 p.m. (EST). E-mail address: docdelivery@haworthpress.com].

are unlikely to engage with the legal system and make their suffering known. Women might also be silenced by fears of violating immigration laws in the United States as well as risking personal loss due to the severe punishment of their partners when indicted by the legal system. *[Article copies available for a fee from The Haworth Document Delivery Service: 1-800-HAWORTH. E-mail address: <docdelivery@haworthpress.com> Website: <http://www.HaworthPress.com> © 2004 by The Haworth Press, Inc. All rights reserved.]*

KEYWORDS. English-speaking Caribbean women, domestic violence, intimate partner violence, Caribbean women, restraining orders, protection orders, Barbados

Perpetrators of abuse who leave an English-speaking Caribbean state like Barbados will find domestic violence laws in many of the states of the United States of America to be more draconian than in their home countries. Although the prosecutorial approach towards domestic violence adapted by many states in the United States is not without fault, perpetrators feel pressured to change their attitudes toward intimate partner violence or face prosecution.

Domestic violence legislation in the United States provides restraining orders for all victims of domestic violence. In states such as Massachusetts and New York, for example, all women qualify for restraining orders as long as they can convince a judge of their present or past engagement in an intimate relationship with a perpetrator of whom they remain fearful. Restraining orders in the United States generally restrict contact between victims and perpetrators rather than encourage reconciliation of partners as legislation in Barbados does (Gondolf 1994; Clarke 1998). If a perpetrator in the United States commits a breach of a restraining order it is customary for the police to arrest that offender. Even when there is no restraining order in effect, police officers in many states in the United States are mandated to arrest perpetrators when they respond to a domestic violence call.

Institutional changes in law enforcement and the court system in many states of the United States have enhanced victims' access to restraining orders. Restraining orders are granted 24 hours each day of the year through judges' authorizations to police officers outside court hours in the United States. The state of Massachusetts established a domestic violence court that deals only with domestic violence cases and provides advocate support to help victims through the legal process. This court, in the past, provided day-care for the children of victims for the duration of court hearings.

Numerous provisions have been made through federal, state and local community resources to assist victims of domestic violence in the United States. Domestic violence shelters across the United States provide a safe haven for women and their children to escape violence. Policy has also been implemented that exempts many domestic violence victims from various requirements in the means-tested welfare system. Nationwide campaigns have been implemented that provide domestic violence victims in the United States with free emergency cell phones and related services that enable battered women to reach someone quickly if they sense immediate danger from their perpetrators. Courts in many states of the United States routinely mandate counseling for male batterers as part of a therapeutic justice response as an alternative to serving jail time (Simon 1995). Perpetrators are routinely expected to pay for such counseling.

Access to restraining orders in the United States has not prevented abuse of women by their intimate partners but it has created an invaluable awareness of the problem and there is evidence that the society treats the problem seriously. Outside of chronic offenders, batterers across the United States are increasingly becoming conscious of and responding to the severity of the provisions of restraining orders. This level of policy awareness is due to the ongoing education of the public, batterers' treatment programs, and supportive services that assist women.

Little is known about how victims of domestic violence from the English-speaking Caribbean fare in the United States. Misconceptions about English-speaking Caribbean immigrants are easily created because of the similarities that this population shares with the African American population (Waters 1999). The dearth of knowledge about English-speaking Caribbean immigrants, and more specifically about domestic violence in this immigrant community, highlights a need to conduct in-depth studies of the experiences of this population.

In lieu of specific knowledge of the experiences of victims of domestic violence from the English-speaking Caribbean states residing in the United States, this study exposes some of the challenges encountered by battered women in the English-speaking Caribbean state of Barbados. The findings of the study are used to support the case that social, cultural and economic factors continue to discourage English-speaking Caribbean women from exercising agency in seeking relief when abused whether in the home countries or as immigrants in the United States.

Close examination of the workings of the Domestic Violence Act, implemented in Barbados in 1992, uncovered the habitual failure of battered women to proactively engage with the legal system. The findings also revealed patterns of behavior among victims and policy implementers that promoted societal indifference toward domestic violence and apathy toward the legislation designed to deter it.

Domestic violence policy may be as helpful as it may be harmful to battered English-speaking Caribbean women at home and abroad. Many negative effects of domestic violence might not be immediately apparent to victims yet the violence can have lasting effects on individuals and the family. Immigrant women from the English-speaking Caribbean who choose not to report abuse and to remain in violent relationships are likely to develop poor mental and physical health conditions. Additionally, women who choose to raise children in violent homes risk their children's positive growth and development. In the final analysis, habitual abusers migrating to the United States risk punishment by a legal system unsympathetic to lower classes, groupings that include many English-speaking Caribbean immigrants (Manning 1996; Buzawa & Buzawa 1996).

DOMESTIC VIOLENCE AND AGENCY

Scholars agree that long acceptance of domestic violence, socioeconomic factors, gender-biased socialization, and asymmetry in relationships promote conflict in Caribbean families (Jordan .1984; Handwerker 1996, 1998; Massiah 1989; Gussler 1996). Conspiracy among family members to protect the family's public image may also protect offenders from punishment and prolong the suffering of victims (Spooner 2001). Police inaction or inappropriate response also raises the risk of repeat abuse (Spooner 2001; Simon 1995).

In societies like the United States problems of racial discrimination and social stigma may further frustrate victims' attempts to seek relief when battered. These factors promote learned helplessness through which battered women narrow their choices to those that they perceive will bring the most positive outcomes (Walker 1993). Women's choices may therefore be perceived by others to be an exhibition of helplessness and poor decision-making in the face of evident danger both in the home country and as immigrants to the United States.

Domestic violence victims, who are most often women, are best served by domestic violence policy when they exercise the power of agency to proactively seek the support of the legal system. Theoretically, agency is important for victims of domestic violence because it represents empowerment to make decisions that are in victims' best interests. Women who make conscious decisions to leave abusive relationships free themselves from victimization and the syndrome of learned helplessness (Walker 1993).

Throughout the literature, agency has been used to represent women's personal decisions to leave abusive relationships (Mahoney 1991, 1994) or more broadly as any action taken to resist violence and through self-determination to regain control and stop abuse (Connell 1997). Battered English-speaking Caribbean women often wish only to calm the home atmosphere or to get immediate and temporary relief from the violence, a concept that is often not understood by persons observing the abuse. To understand battered women's reluctance to seek assistance, it is important to frame women's dilemma in the context of women's action that may not be finite or lucid because of an unresponsive and complex legal system, and social and economic constraints (Lazarus-Black 2001).

LOCUS OF THE STUDY–BARBADOS

Barbados, the locus of this study, is one of the larger English-speaking Caribbean islands. The independent island state–430 sq km in size–lies at the extreme east of the Caribbean island chain. In 1996 the Barbados population was estimated to be 264,595 (Report on Vital Statistics and Registrations for 1996, Barbados Registration Department, Supreme Court, Barbados).

Sporadic economic growth and economic troubles from the 1970s through the 1990s, promoted annual unemployment rates in the Barbados economy that often exceeded 10% (Duncan 1994). Structural adjustment policies further rend the fabric of the society contributing to excessive public indigence, illegal drug use and violence among residents (Duncan 1994). Steady growth of the population and ongoing out migration of the economically active population have placed pressure on the government to provide additional social services with limited state budgets. Fiscal asceticism has become imperative in an economy showing only modest success in its economic diversification plan (Duncan 1994).

High literacy rates among the Barbados population–estimated in 1991 to be 91%–can be attributed to the state's provision of free compulsory education from age five to 16 years (Mohammed & Perkins 1999). This well-educated work force is, however, deeply stratified with women engaging primarily in domestic services and men in higher paying professional and trade occupations. The strong religious beliefs of the Barbados population are mostly embedded in practices of the Church of England (Mohammed & Perkins 1999). Recent growth in evangelical ministries has seen an upsurge in church membership. Clergy and apostles of the various religious denominations in Barbados educate their flock in doctrine that promotes commitment to marriage and male household headship premised on scriptural authority. Beyond reinforcing male authority in the home, much of the religious instruction fails to proactively address women's subjugation and abuse by their intimate partners.

Registered marriages in Barbados fluctuated from 1995 until 1998 while divorce petitions have increased annually. The number of marriages registered in Barbados increased slightly two years in succession during the period 1995 and 1996 but fell in 1997 and rose again in 1998. Growing divorce rates together with the prevalence of long-term visiting relationships contributed to a 43.5% rate of female-headed households in Barbados (Mohammed & Perkins 1999). Women initiated the majority of divorces in Barbados where divorce petitions average 12 per 100 marriages annually and in 1998 totaled 510 (Report on Vital Statistics and Registrations for 1998, Registration Department, Supreme Court, Barbados). The matrifocal structure of Barbados families supports the raising of children by women while encouraging men to spend extended periods of time socializing with other males outside the home. In some instances, men's contribution to family life is limited to exertion of power and control through violence against their mates and children (Handwerker 1998).

The Barbados Supreme Court oversees the legal system in Barbados, a system not well-understood and utilized by the Barbadian citizenry. The legal system in Barbados comprises Magistrates' Courts where magistrates, without a jury, conduct cases quickly and with less formality, the High Court, and the Court of Appeal that comprise the Supreme Court. Hence, the legal system becomes a course of last resort for domestic violence victims in Barbados. Women's fear of humiliation in the courts has kept many victims from seeking restraining orders (Clarke 1998). In 1998, 494 restraining order applications were lodged by a variety of household members, under the Domestic Violence Act Cap. 130 in the Barbados courts. Applications in previous years totaled 419 cases in 1997, 266 cases in 1996, 109 in 1995, and nine cases in 1994 (Report on Vital Statistics and Registrations for 1998, Registration Department, Supreme Court, Barbados). Poor monitoring of the legislation made it impossible to determine the number of restraining orders granted since the law was enacted.

Policymakers in Barbados face the challenge of addressing a social problem with limited resources in a culture that is strongly patriarchal in nature. Social problems like domestic violence compete with development and maintenance of the economic infrastructure for scarce resources. The lack of adequate economic resources negatively affects the state's ability to provide ancillary support services that would enhance the effectiveness of the domestic violence legislation. Deeply embedded cultural practices and beliefs among the Barbados population also discourage victims from seeking relief while raising the level of hostility toward the legislation and backlash against women, particularly among men.

INVADING A MAN'S CASTLE

Passage of the Barbados domestic violence legislation repulsed many Barbadian men who were aware of the legislation's provisions. The Barbados Domestic Violence (Restraining orders) legislation is part of a broader effort by policymakers in Barbados to shore up family rights. This effort has been ongoing since the island's independence in 1966 with legislative reform in areas such as succession, the status of children and right of abode.

A major concern among opponents of the Domestic Violence Act was that for the first time in the history of this independent state, the culturally sacred space of the home was to be invaded by the state. The terms of the legislation made it " . . . frightening that so much of normal behavior hallowed by long acceptance should suddenly be criminalized by this piece of legislation" (Mr. L. R. Tull, Official Report, House of Assembly Debates, First Session 1991-1996, p. 165). In opposition to the policy it was argued " . . . the state has no business in the bedroom of the nation. You cannot have Government going into people's bedrooms and that is at the heart of the philosophy of our position" (Mr. L. R. Tull, Official Report, House of Assembly Debates, First Session 1991-1996, p. 163).

Popular belief that the home is beyond the reach of the law, presents a major obstacle in addressing domestic violence in English-speaking Caribbean states like Barbados.

> The same culture of which I speak, Mr. Speaker, says that a man's home is his castle. I do not care how much legislation you import from Britain, you have to deal with a mental cultural mindset before you rush into this kind of legislation because the last state is likely to be worse than the first. (Mr. L. R. Tull, Official Report, House of Assembly Debates, First Session 1991-1996, p. 163)

The decision by policymakers to implement restraining orders in a growing number of English-speaking Caribbean states has not convinced opponents of governments' right to use whatever means might be necessary to protect victims of domestic violence. Many cynics continue to challenge policy by affirming that the government should not manage people's behavior in the privacy of the home. Smith (1996) posits, "It is not for the state to dictate how people should behave in their private lives, and one may doubt the degree to which professional intervention should be used in family affairs" (Smith 1996, p. 455)

In the culturally male-dominant societies of the English-speaking Caribbean the real effect of domestic violence legislation has not been felt. For many observers in the Caribbean societies,

> Legislation doesn't mean a thing, it's just pen and paper. The average guy in his home doesn't care and when he's in a state of anger he's going to beat his woman. Most men aren't aware of the laws but in a moment of passion they don't care. (Tony Robinson, Jamaican columnist, quoted by Barnes 2000)

Domestic violence in the English-speaking Caribbean as in other jurisdictions globally remains a complex issue. Activists like Penelope Beckles, attorney-at-law and president of the Rape Crisis Centre in Trinidad and Tobago argue,

> Domestic violence is a complex, multifaceted phenomenon which is international in scope and destructive to the fabric of society. It requires a multi-sectoral approach involving government, private and international agencies, as well as non-governmental and community legislative and non-legislative types in every aspect of life. (Barnes 2000, IPS)

PROTECTING VICTIMS IN BARBADOS

The task of protecting domestic violence victims is complex. Legislative reform removes some obstacles but also presents additional challenges in the policy environment. Prior to the passage of the domestic violence legislation in Barbados, perpetrators of domestic violence were tried under criminal law in the same manner as stranger crimes. Under these provisions cases took long periods of time to be heard by magistrates if ever they were prosecuted.

Perpetrators of simple assault, assault and battery, and other misdemeanors against their intimate partners were usually warned by police officers. More serious offenses such as wounding with intent to commit bodily harm were more likely to be prosecuted and punished by jail time and/or fines upon indictment. Perpetrators indicted of murder or manslaughter risked capital punishment or a lifetime sentence.

Under the provisions of traditional criminal law police officers in Barbados called upon to stop domestic violence faced several challenges. Acts of domestic violence were treated as stranger crimes if the decision was not arbitrarily made by officers to overlook domestic violence incidents as "family matters" that fell outside the jurisdiction of the criminal law. "The abuse suffered primarily by women and children in the family and intimate relationships has been generally invisible in law–it was labeled a private matter, best addressed by the family and inappropriate for legal resolution" (Robinson 1999).

The Barbados domestic violence legislation changed the provisions, if not the actual outcomes, for victims of domestic violence. The policy, although coached in mediatory terms, represents a significant and progressive approach to domestic violence by policymakers in the island state of Barbados.

Recent legislative reform in Barbados introduced the potential for victims of domestic violence to seek speedy relief before the law and for magistrates to punish perpetrators of abuse in ways that were previously impossible. Major tenets of the legislation made provision for victims and their representatives to approach the court for restraining orders. The legislation granted magistrates the powers to exclude domestic violence perpetrators from the home and to prevent them from stalking or harassing their mates. Perpetrators, given notice of an issue of restraining order with arrest, risk serving one year in prison, a fine of $5,000 or both for breach of such order (Barbados Domestic Violence [Restraining orders] Act 1992). At the same time, the domestic violence legislation empowers magistrates to reduce the severity of punishment of breadwinners who promise to refrain from repeat abuse.

Magistrates in Barbados are most likely to recommend mandatory counseling or to restrict proximity of perpetrators to their victims or their involvement of third parties in harassing such victims. Only under extraneous circumstances do magistrates separate couples in violent relationships. Lenient punishment of perpetrators results from a complex combination of limitations in the crafting of the Barbados domestic violence legislation but also from the culture of the people of Barbados. For example, the Barbados domestic violence legislation requires that magistrates uphold the institution of the family in decisions in domestic violence cases. No provisions are made to protect women in visiting relationships within the legislation because the legislation applies only to cohabiting couples. In a society where a significant number of couples engage in intimate relations without living together, it is easy to see how the effectiveness of the Barbados domestic violence legislation might be easily compromised.

METHODOLOGY

In an attempt to understand how effective the Barbados Domestic Violence (Protection Orders) Act of 1992 might have been in protecting battered women, 368 police records of domestic violence were examined. The records, dated from 1994 to 1998, were extracted from the vaults of three police stations located in the suburbs of Bridgetown, the capital of Barbados. Reports selected for this study were made by wives, ex-wives, girlfriends, and ex-girlfriends. The content of procedural hearings conducted in magistrates' courts in Bridgetown and interviews with 19 battered women–seven with restraining orders–several domestic violence advocates, police officers and legal personnel were also included in the study.

FINDINGS

Women's power of agency in seeking relief may be frustrated by cultural and economic factors. Victims' reliance on their perpetrators for economic support or unreasonable opportunity costs reduces the probability of prosecution of abusers (Ford 1991; Fagan 1996; Jordan 1986; Spooner 2001). In a legal system that appears to have shifted little to accommodate the functioning of Barbados' recently implemented restraining orders legislation, one police officer observed that,

> Women also don't want to go to court because the process is too long. They may have to go to court five or six times before the case is heard. A woman may go to court and spend all day to be told that she has to come back on another date. Women say they have to lose a day's pay at work and they cannot afford to do so. That has a lot to do with government–we need magistrates to deal with the backlog of cases. (Police Officer, Royal Barbados Police Force)

Women's attempts to exercise agency might also be diverted by skepticism and lack of confidence in the legal system. Qualified women who approach the court in Barbados do not necessarily find immediate relief. The women interviewed waited for anywhere from three days to one week for a hearing and subsequently to secure restraining orders. Women are therefore constantly seeking alternatives to the legal system to address their problems. One woman interviewed described the orders as "a waste of time, a piece of paper cannot protect you." Another did not believe that the order would deter her spouse from abusing her and stated instead her wish to "get a sharp-edged weapon and slice off his hand." Yet another woman felt that church attendance and a Christian outlook on life would be more beneficial than "airing dirty linen in public" by seeking a restraining order.

Women in Barbados may seek police assistance only to bring immediate peace to the household, hence the numerous requests in police files asking that police officers warn their abusers. Victims often have no interest in long-term engagement with the legal system nor do they perceive their actions to be part of a greater plan to claim their rights (Walker 1993). Spooner (2001) found that more women in her study sought relief–whether from family, the police, legal system or private agencies–when they perceived the abuse to be severe.

Police officers and advocates for battered women interviewed for this study linked police reluctance to arrest and prosecute perpetrators to women's reluctance to follow through with legal charges against perpetrators. The police in Barbados generally acquiesce to requests not to prosecute perpetrators. It is unclear whether this is done to purge the system of cases that might not be indictable or because of habitual practices in implementing criminal law. This report in the police records depicts this.

> Boyfriend and father of two children. She wants him warned against beating her. He was interviewed and admitted to hitting her, saying, she would not listen to him when he speaks to her. He was warned against ill-treating or beating [*Complainant*]. He said "OK Officer." However, [*Complainant*] was advised in accordance with the Domestic Violence Act and she stated she does not require prosecution against offender.

The following case of domestic violence documented in police records was not uncommon either through reports or anecdotal evidence from key informants.

> [*Alleged offender*] was seen at shop. He was very aggressive and appeared to be under the influence of alcohol. He was reminded that there is a restraining order enforced by the magistrate . . . which prevents him from beating, threatening or harassing [*Complainant*] and was advised against breaching this restraining order. He replied "Man, I ain't even wanta hear wunnuh. I ain't got nothing to say to wunnuh."

Why might a police officer be reluctant to arrest an offender who admits to violence against his partner? Why might an officer not arrest an offender who is clearly in violation of a restraining order? Not unlike the response of the legal system in the United States until recently, domestic violence cases in Barbados' legal system receive low priority. Only women who are persistent are likely to achieve success in prosecuting their perpetrators. Numerous cases of abuse reported to the police since the implementation of the Barbados domestic violence legislation have resulted in perpetrators being warned and victims referred for medical care if physical injury is observed. The following police report presents such a situation.

> [*Complainant*], her boyfriend and two children have been living at the same address for the past seven years. The complainant and her boyfriend have been together for 13 years. As a result of their relationship, [*the complainant*] became the mother of [*the alleged offender's*] daughter, 12 years. She has another daughter 13 years. For the past 13 years they have been having disputes and domestic problems. During the past

three years of the relationship she was injured by him on her right shoulder and she left him. He then made several calls requesting her to return to him for another two years and then left and went living with a female friend. In 1988 [*the complainant*] and the two children moved to the present home. Since then they have been having quarrels and fights and the services of the police was requested. [*the alleged offender's*] behavio[u]r has not changed towards the complainant and her children. On Saturday . . . about 0825 hours the complainant, [*the alleged offender*] and two children were at home. The complainant was standing at the back door when [*the alleged offender*] took a bowl of water and throw it out the back door but before the complainant could move out of the door properly some of the water went on her. She took the mat at the door and dried up the water. The complainant was in the area of the said back door when [the alleged offender] returned with another bowl of water, as he turned to speak to her he slip on the mat hurting his foot in the process. [*The alleged offender*] then throw the second bowl of water at the complainant, she moved her head to avoid being struck. [*the alleged offender*] then took up a broomstick, charged at the complainant and strike her across her left foot below her knee and on her left hand. She rushed into the bedroom hurting her back in the process. [*the alleged offender*] continued charging at the complainant. She then ran out of the house for safety. She was interviewed and given a medical condition form to seek medical attention.

Despite this victim's qualification for a restraining order, no record was made by the police of referring the victim to the court for such an order. There was no arrest of this abuser, nor of the abusers in the previous cited cases, although the report indicates that because of previous incidents of violence the police knew the parties. Clearly, the police treated these cases of domestic violence as they have customarily done under criminal law, by referring physically impaired victims for medical assistance without seeking to prosecute or further punish offenders.

Battered women in Barbados may not always receive sympathetic hearings before magistrates. One police officer blamed some magistrates for treating battered women as if they were villains. Magistrates' rulings, to a large extent, place the responsibility for couples' resolution outside the ambit of the criminal court. Discussions with magistrates of the Bridgetown magistrates' courts as well as clerical officers of the courts indicated a clear preference for sending couples to counseling rather than issuing restraining orders or separating perpetrator and victim. One magistrate expressed the opinion that legally married couples are better served by the counsel of clergy given that the church endowed the vows of marriage.

Magistrates' rulings in domestic violence hearings are often an intricate combination of magistrates' perceptions that women wish to remain in relationships as well as the limitations of the domestic violence legislation. Magistrates are forced to ponder serious questions. Should the need to keep a family intact override the safety of family members? What conditions are serious enough to warrant an abusive partner leaving the home for a victim's safety without threatening the stability of the institution of the family?

Section 7 (c) of the Barbados Domestic Violence Act 1992 limits the ambit of magistrates by the requirement, among other things, that the court considers the "need to preserve and protect the institution of marriage or a union other than marriage and to give protection and assistance to the family as a natural and fundamental group unit in society" (p. 10). This value coupled with direct orders for mandatory counseling serves a goal other than that of restraining orders legislation in the United States, which is to separate victim and perpetrator. This outcome is not unlike that encountered in the early stages of implementation of domestic violence legislation in the United States (Ptacek 1999).

Caribbean women are reluctant participants in court processes due to fears of public humiliation (Clarke 1998; Gussler 1996). The Barbados population generally, and women in particular, have limited experience in seeking rights before the law without legal counsel. Yet the Barbados legislation provides no advocate support for victims and only limited attempts have been made to restructure the legal process to remove the hindrances that may deter women from seeking refuge in the legal system.

Unlike the provision of domestic violence legislation in the United States that provides relief for all women who are or were in a substantial intimate relationship, qualified women in Barbados must be in co-habiting relationships with their abusers to qualify for relief under the domestic violence legislation. For a significant number of Barbadian women, therefore, the domestic violence legislation provides no relief. Women in Barbados are unable to routinely acquire restraining orders on a 24-hour basis. Unlike the system in place in many states in the United States where women access restraining orders around the clock (Jaffe et al. 1996), restraining orders are only available in Barbados during the hours that courts are open: 8 a.m. to 4 p.m., Monday to Friday and a half day on Saturdays. These practices might prevent immigrant English-speaking Caribbean women in the United States from applying for restraining orders if they are unaware of the variations in the provisions of domestic violence legislation in the United States.

CONCLUSIONS

Inherent weaknesses aside, the Barbados domestic violence legislation represents one of the most advanced legal responses to domestic violence among

English-speaking Caribbean states. Its provisions enable battered women to prosecute their abusers without intervention by a third party, ending centuries of reliance on the police or legal counsel to plead on their behalf. The legislation also has the potential, with amendments, to encourage women's agency in seeking their rights whether in their home country or in countries such as the United States.

Despite the implementation of the Barbados domestic violence legislation, battered women have not reaped the overwhelming benefits that the policy promises. Women remain reluctant to appear before the court to settle domestic violence cases for fear of humiliation by the legal system and subsequent economic loss. In a cultural environment where women remain silent about domestic violence, often seeking the assistance of police or other agencies only when the abuse is severe, many women suffer violence to protect the family's image. Ineffective police response to domestic violence also contributes to women's skepticism about the ability of the legal system to protect them from repeat abuse.

Women in Barbados most often exercise agency not as an exit or permanent severance from a relationship but, on repeated occasions, to manage the violence. For many women, exiting a relationship means a loss of social status, a home and the security it provides. Therefore their implementation of agency is more in line with Connell's (1997) concept of agency as resistance in any form that would stop the abuse and enable control. In lieu of trust in the legal system, the majority of women in Barbados silently draw on their religious belief and faith in God to protect them from violence and to change the lives of their batterers. Several of the women interviewed in Barbados cherished the belief that things would improve if only their partners would "attend church and have a Christian outlook on life." In many ways this is the most that some women feel empowered to do since women have not fully grasped the concept of seeking their rights before the law as women have in the United States.

Even if English-speaking Caribbean women were to overcome their cultural reservations and seek the assistance of the legal system, significant, institutional and systemic barriers such as fear of racial discrimination, deportation or the social services system remain. Battered English-speaking Caribbean women seeking to exercise agency in escaping violence must therefore be cautious. Despite the array of services available to victims of domestic violence in the United States, battered English-speaking Caribbean immigrants may still be at a disadvantage, for example, in seeking relief from the legal system. In the United States, complex immigration laws govern the status of immigrants. Women may be denied access to resources under the stipulations of the Illegal Immigration Reform and Immigrant Responsibility Act (IIRIRA).

In 1996 the United States Congress passed the Illegal Immigration Reform and Immigrant Responsibility Act (IIRIRA). The Act placed severe restrictions on family-based immigration, introduced "removal" and its related due process in deportation cases as well as depriving the federal courts of the right to review unlawful decisions by INS officers and immigration judges. Virtually all of the public benefits for immigrants were additionally removed with the passage of the 1996 "welfare reform" bill. Though some benefits were bestowed on immigrant women with the passage of the Violence Against Women Act (VAWA) in 1994 with its broad provisions for immigrant victims of domestic violence, the outcomes for battered immigrant women are still indeterminable. Under such conditions battered women might fail to seek relief for fear of deportation.

Policymakers in the United States seeking to assist battered immigrant women from the English-speaking Caribbean should be aware that cultural, social and economic factors are likely to interact in ways that create harmful outcomes for them. Since the majority of English-speaking Caribbean immigrants are black, they are likely to be treated with the same prejudice and injustice in the legal system as the African American population in the United States. English-speaking Caribbean families might find that they are increasingly targeted by the legal system for negative treatment. "Because arrests in domestic violence disputes are disproportionately of lower class, minority residents of large cities (Buzawa & Buzawa, 1990), the policy extracts yet an additional cost, or 'crime tariff' (Packer, 1965), from them. Not all families are being policed for 'violence' " (Manning 1996, p. 92).

Good intentions to protect English-speaking Caribbean women from intimate violence in the United States may impact couples negatively. Women who are pressured to prosecute their intimate partners might develop a sense of betrayal of their partners and extended family relationships (Stark 1996). English-speaking Caribbean males will find the legal system in the United States responds in starkly different ways than they routinely experience in their home country. Cases of domestic violence that may be overlooked in the English-speaking Caribbean bring severe punishment such as the possibility of serving jail time in the United States. In a legal system, guided by prejudice and unwilling to negotiate or to be ignored, immigrant English-speaking Caribbean men who are indicted of domestic violence offenses, face the risk of deportation and its resultant economic hardships for their partners and children.

Given the lack of knowledge about the experiences of battered immigrant women from the English-speaking Caribbean in the United States, significant contributions can be made to the literature through future research among this population. Areas of specific research include development of an understanding of women's experiences in the legal system when they report incidents of domestic violence to the police. It would be important to understand the extent to which women do turn to the police and subsequently the rate of incarceration of domestic violence perpetrators from the English-speaking Caribbean as a result of women's reports to the police.

Future policymaking should be focused on educating English-speaking Caribbean women about their rights while drawing on their strong coping and resiliency. Spooner (2001) posits that women in Barbados control the state's intrusion into their lives by reporting only serious incidents of abuse to the police. Great confidence is instead placed in family and friends, churches and, to a lesser extent, social agencies. Policymakers and activists in the United States can help battered women from English-speaking Caribbean countries by supporting and strengthening women's informal social networks, settings in which women share and support each other. Churches in the immigrant communities are also important outreach centers through which various types of services might reach women. Understanding that the experiences, needs, and in some instances, aspirations of English-speaking Caribbean immigrants differ from those of the African American population, is key to connecting with women from English-speaking Caribbean countries. Strong advocacy support in navigating the court and legal system in the United States is vital in empowering English-speaking Caribbean women to exercise agency to seek relief from domestic violence.

REFERENCES

Barnes, Corinne, 1 June 2000 Despite legislation, violence against women continues–*http://www.hartford-hwp.com/archives/43/116.html*-Article No. 97563).

Buzawa, E. & Buzawa, C. G. (1996). *Do arrests and restraining orders work?* Thousand Oaks: Sage Publications.

Chaney, C.K. & Saltzstein, G.H. (1998). Democratic control and bureaucratic responsiveness: The police and domestic violence. *American Journal of Political Science*, Vol. 42, No. 3, 745-768.

Clarke, R. (1998). *Violence against women in the Caribbean: State and non-state responses.* New York: UNIFEM.

Connell, P. (1997). Understanding victimization and agency. Considerations of race, class and gender. *Political and Legal Anthropology Review*, 20(2), 115-143.

Domestic Violence (Restraining orders) Act, 1992. CAP.130A. Laws of Barbados.

Duncan, N. (1994). Barbados: Democracy at the crossroads. In C.J. Edie (Ed.), *Democracy in the Caribbean: Myths and realities.* Westport, CT: Praeger.

Fagan, J. (1996). The criminalization of domestic violence: Promises and limits. Paper presented at the 1995 Conference on Criminal Justice Research and Evaluation. Washington, DC.

Fine, D.M. (1998). The Violence Against Women Act of 1994: The proper federal role in policing domestic violence. *Cornell Law Review*, Vol. 84, 252-303.

Gondolf, E. W. (1994). Court responses to petitions for civil restraining orders. *Journal of Interpersonal Violence*, 9(4), 503-516.

Gussler, J. (1996). Adaptive strategies and social networks of women in St. Kitts. In C. Barrow (Ed.), *Family in the Caribbean: Themes and perspectives* (pp. 119-134). Ian Randle Publishers, Kingston; James Currey Publishers, Oxford: Marcus Wiener Publishers.

Handwerker, W.P. (1996). Power and gender: Violence and affection experienced by children in Barbados, West Indies. *Medical Anthropology*, 17, 101-128.

Handwerker, W.P. (1998). Why violence? A test of hypotheses representing three discourses on the roots of domestic violence. *Human Organization*, 57, No. 2, 200-208.

Jaffe, P.G., Lemon, N.K.D., Sandler, J., & Wolfe, D.A. (1996). *Working together to end domestic violence*. Tampa FL: Mancorp Publishing Inc.

Jordan, M. (1986). *Physical violence against women in Barbados*. Barbados Bureau of Women's Affairs.

Lazarus-Black, M. (2001). Law and the pragmatics of inclusion: Governing domestic violence in Trinidad and Tobago. *American Ethnologist*, 28(2), 388-416.

Mahoney, M.R. (1994). Victimization or Oppression? Women's lives, violence and agency. In Martha Albertson Fineman & Roxanne Mykitiuk (Eds.), *The public nature of private violence: The discovery of domestic abuse* (pp. 59-92).

Manning, P.K. (1996). The preventive conceit. The black box in market context. In E. S. Buzawa & C.G. Buzawa (Eds.), *Do arrests and restraining orders work?* Thousand Oaks, London, New Delhi: Sage Publications.

Massiah, J. (1989). Women's lives and livelihoods: A view from the Commonwealth Caribbean. *World Development*, 17, 979-991.

Mohammed, P. & Perkins, A. (1999). *Caribbean women at the crossroads. The paradox of motherhood among women of Barbados, St. Lucia and Dominica. Barbados, Jamaica, Trinidad and Tobago*. Canoe Press, University of the West Indies.

National Institute of Justice (1990). *Civil restraining orders: Legislation, current court practice, and enforcement*. Washington, DC: U.S. Department of Justice.

Official Report, Barbados House of Assembly Debates, First Session 1991-1996.

Ptacek, J. (1999). *Battered women in the courtroom. The power of judicial responses*. Boston: Northeaster University Press.

Report on Vital Statistics and Registrations for 1996. Registration Department, Supreme Court, Barbados.

Report on Vital Statistics and Registrations for 1998. Registration Department, Supreme Court, Barbados.

Robinson, T. (1999). Changing conceptions of violence: The impact of domestic violence legislation in the Caribbean. *The Caribbean Law Review*, Vol. 9, No. 1, 113-135.

Simon, L. M. J. (1995). A therapeutic jurisprudence approach to the legal processing of domestic violence cases. *Psychology, Public Policy and Law*, Vol. 1, No. 1, 43-79.

Smith, R.T. (1996). Family, social change and social policy in the West Indies. In C. Barrow (Ed.), *Family in the Caribbean: Themes and perspectives* (pp. 440-455). Kingston: Ian Randle Publishers.

Spooner, M. (2001). Women under subjection of the law: A study of the legal responses to women's abuse in the English-speaking Caribbean. Unpublished Ph.D. dissertation, University of Massachusetts Boston, Boston, MA.

Stark, E. (1996). Mandatory arrest of batterers: A reply to critics. In E.S. Buzawa & C.G. Buzawa (Eds.), *Do arrests and restraining orders work?* Thousand Oaks, London, New Delhi: Sage Publications.

Walker, Lenore A. (1993). The battered woman syndrome is a psychological consequence of abuse. In R.J. Gelles & D.R. Loseke (Eds.), *Current controversies on family violence* (pp. 133-153). Newbury Park, London, Delhi: Sage Publication.

Waters, M.C. (1999). *Black identities: West Indian immigrant dreams and American realities*. Cambridge MA and London, England: Harvard University Press.

Social Work with West Indian Fa
A Multilevel Approach

Carol Ann Daniel

SUMMARY. This conceptual analysis explores the psychosocial and cultural experiences of English-speaking West Indians in the United States. Relevant factors include family role changes; parent/child conflicts; prolonged separation from and reunification with parents; finding suitable employment and education-related issues. The challenge for social work is to develop programs for these families that contribute to their social and economic integration. Given the extent to which social, economic and related policies impact on the needs of this population, the author suggests that a multilevel approach which utilizes the micro skills associated with individual intervention and the macro strategies of intervening at the societal and institutional levels is needed. This approach necessarily includes activities such as advocacy and empowerment. *[Article copies available for a fee from The Haworth Document Delivery Service: 1-800-HAWORTH. E-mail address: <docdelivery@haworthpress.com> Website: <http://www. HaworthPress.com> © 2004 by The Haworth Press, Inc. All rights reserved.]*

KEYWORDS. West Indians, immigration, families, social work practice, advocacy and empowerment

Carol Ann Daniel, CSW, ABD, is Assistant Professor of Sociology at Brooklyn College, City University of New York.

[Haworth co-indexing entry note]: "Social Work with West Indian Families: A Multilevel Approach." Daniel, Carol Ann. Co-published simultaneously in *Journal of Immigrant & Refugee Services* (The Haworth Social Work Practice Press, an imprint of The Haworth Press, Inc.) Vol. 2, No. 3/4, 2004, pp. 135-145; and: *The Health and Well-Being of Caribbean Immigrants in the United States* (ed: Annette M. Mahoney) The Haworth Social Work Practice Press, an imprint of The Haworth Press, Inc., 2004, pp. 135-145. Single or multiple copies of this article are available for a fee from The Haworth Document Delivery Service [1-800-HAWORTH. 9:00 a.m. - 5:00 p.m. (EST). E-mail address: docdelivery@haworthpress.com].

The process of migration means both fulfillment and hardship for many immigrants as they attempt to meet the demands of urban life and adjust to an alien culture. Many of the problems they encounter arise from their interaction with the environment and involve social, economic and political factors. Efforts by social work to work with immigrants have tended to focus more on their cultural adaptation and, in particular, developing an understanding of how practice can be sensitive to differences in the worldviews of immigrants (Padilla, 1997). However, social workers working with West Indian immigrants are faced with a complex array of issues requiring specific knowledge about their culture and the psychosocial processes and effects associated with migration.

The social work practice literature on working with West Indian families is relatively sparse. A review of the literature reveals that this population faces a series of stress-producing events that often results in the need for social work services. Intervention may be necessary due to problems in the parent/child relationship, family role changes, and employment and education-related difficulties (Mahoney, 2002; Thrasher and Anderson, 1988; McNicol, 1993; Sowell-Coker et al., 1985). The literature also reveals that this population has low service utilization rates. These low rates have been attributed to cultural insensitivity among service providers in understanding their values and life-styles, lack of knowledge and experience in using services, and reluctance to receive assistance outside of the family (Thrasher and Anderson, 1988; McNicol, 1993; Sowell-Coker et al., 1985; Mathews, 1994; Smith and Mason, 1995).

Most families who come in contact with social workers and other human service providers do so through referrals by school personnel and child protective services as a result of suspected child abuse or neglect (Thrasher and Anderson, 1988; McNicol, 1993). For those who are self-referred, school-related problems are identified as the primary source of conflict and the identified client is usually a child (Sowell-Coker et al., 1985; McNicol, 1993; Thrasher and Anderson, 1988).

This paper discusses various aspects of the psychosocial and cultural experience of West Indian immigrant families in the United States and the impact on their social functioning. They include family relationships, child-rearing practices, separation from and reunification with parents and other potential sources of family conflict associated with immigration. A multilevel approach aimed at increasing their ability to create individual and community change is also discussed.

FAMILY RELATIONSHIPS

The West Indian family structure is multi-generational consisting of the nuclear family, grandparents, aunts and uncles (Thrasher and Anderson, 1988; McNicol, 1993). There is also data suggesting that the large number of female-headed households mirrors those prevailing in the Caribbean. For example, Grasmuck and Grosfoguel (1997) found that the percentage of female-headed households for Jamaicans in New York City is 33% and 34% in Jamaica.

Within the husband-wife/partner relationship there is a pattern of gender-differentiated roles and activities. Women assume most of the responsibilities for household labor, and fathers are designated as the main provider. As the head of household, a man's primary role within the family is one of economic support for his wife and children. In contrast, a woman's primary role is that of child rearing which includes socialization and discipline (Sowell-Coker, 1985; McNicol, 1993; Roopnarine and Brown, 1997). The extended family also plays a significant role by providing emotional and financial support to both the parents and the children (Brice, 1982).

CHILD REARING PRACTICES

West Indian parents often use a parenting style that is authoritarian and punitive (Baptiste et al., 1997). The goal is obedience and respect from children at all times. Those who fail to comply with these expectations may be slapped, beaten with a belt or strap, and spanked (Payne, 1989; McNicol, 1993; Sowell-Coker et al., 1985). Moreover, while Americans emphasize self-reliance and independence, West Indians place little importance on these values. Therefore expressions of assertion or independence are often seen as disrespectful and are considered as grounds for punishment.

In a study conducted of 449 West Indian parents, respondents identified corporal punishment as a deterrent to future behavior, and as a tool to instill discipline, respect for parents and obedience (Payne, 1989). The findings of McNicol (1993) and Thrasher and Anderson (1988) support Payne's (1993) conclusions that West Indian parents endorse corporal punishment as the most effective means of controlling children's behavior and instilling respect for elders. However, as Baker (1993) points out, physical punishment does little to control children's behavior and may have negative effects on their development. For example, by relying on physical punishment as the primary means of discipline, ideas of right and wrong may not be internalized or reasoned, but compliance may depend more on the circumstances, such as the presence of people recognized as powerful.

As they witness the assertiveness and independence of American children, West Indian children often become resentful of their parents' authoritarian behavior and rigid controls. Baptiste et al., (1997) as cited in Roopnarine and Brown, 1997) suggest that children's rebellion may also be attributed to ethnic identity confusion in the new culture, adjusting to school and disappointment with parents' ability to provide a more successful life in the new society. However, parents often see their rebellion as a threat to the family structure and a desertion of important family values. As children rebel and become disobedient some parents may also succumb to despair and depression. Others are investigated and their children removed from the home due to allegations of child abuse and neglect (McNicol, 1993; Sowell-Coker et al., 1985; Thrasher and Anderson, 1988; Baptiste et al., 1997). When parents are confronted with allegations of child abuse they are often angry and confused that their belief in physical punishment as an appropriate method of child rearing was in conflict with the values of the dominant culture (Thrasher and Anderson, 1988).

SEPARATION FROM AND REUNIFICATION WITH PARENTS

In addition to issues around discipline and adjusting to the new culture, some of the greatest difficulties arise when children are separated from their parents for long periods of time and their subsequent reunification. Several authors have noted that a significant number of West Indian parents who migrate to the U.S. leave their children behind in their home country (Arnold, 1997; Sowell-Coker et al., 1985; Palmer, 1995; McNicol, 1993; Thrasher and Anderson, 1988; Soto, 1987). More recent migration patterns indicate that women are migrating first since there are usually better opportunities for them to find employment (Kasinitz and Vickerman, 2001; McNicol, 1993; Arnold, 1997).

During her absence the children are cared for by a member of the extended family with the expectation that they will be united once she has established herself in the new country. This temporary transferral of parental rights is commonly referred to as child fostering and is widely practiced among West Indians (Soto, 1987). For example, in a study of 30 West Indian immigrants Thrasher and Anderson (1988) reported that all of the adults immigrated alone without their spouse or children and that 76% of the children were raised by people other than their biological parents. However, the separation and subsequent reunification years later often present psychological difficulties for children. For instance, most of the children become bonded with the person who cared for them in their parent's absence. As such, they may go through a period of mourning for the people they left behind. Mahoney (2002) notes that relocation disrupts the structures of emotional and social support that are necessary for children's psychological well-being further complicating their adjustment. Others (Roopnarine and Brown, 1997) suggest that some of the difficulties children experience may have their origins first in the disruption of the bond to a primary attachment figure at a sensitive period in the child's life, and again with the termination of relationships with individuals who cared for the child during the parental absence. Mahoney (2002) suggests that for adolescents the stresses of migration can be especially problematic as it can further complicate their search for identity. When this happens, previously unresolved issues of trust, initiative, industry and identity reemerge making the adolescent vulnerable to social and academic problems.

Apart from the grief of separation, some children become confused and resentful in finding themselves in a new environment with people they barely know or remember. Some rebel by running away while others withdraw. Still others reject their parents by looking to previous caretakers in the home country for guidance.

The long separation not only creates problems for children but for their parents as well. Many parents become disappointed and angry when their children appear withdrawn or unhappy by their reunion. Others may have missed the formative years in their children's lives and are challenged to integrate them into the family in the new society (Sowell-Coker et al., 1985; McNicol, 1993; Thrasher and Anderson, 1988).

OTHER SOURCES OF FAMILY CONFLICT/STRESS

Employment

In addition to the aforementioned problems, West Indian immigrants also experience several important life circumstances that also put them at risk for social work services. They include employment problems, family role changes, and problems with the education system.

Most West Indians migrate to the United States for economic reasons (Palmer, 1995). As such, they are highly motivated to improve the quality of life for themselves and their relatives back home. Consequently, many are willing to take any work available to them including some of the hardest and most menial work. However, the low wages and financial insecurity that accompany poor employment often mean that they must work more than one job in order to achieve their goals. This pattern of employment often results in family conflicts as it allows little time for personal and family interactions.

Family conflicts are further increased as those men for whom migration has meant a loss of status try more forcefully to command the respect and authority that is denied them both at work and in the larger society (McNicol, 1993). McNicol (1993) observed that some men experience even greater displacement when they are unable to find work while their wives can. Problems may also arise as the new economic independence of the wife clashes with the traditional expectations of the husband (Bonnett, 1990 as cited in Palmer, 1995). Thus, at a time when they most need the security and support from their families, many West Indians find their family relations changed which can be a source of great stress and extreme pain.

Education

In addition to their strong work ethic, West Indians value education highly, as they believe it is the only way of achieving upward mobility and a better way of life (Sowell-Coker et al., 1985) As a result, they are often anxious for their children to do well in school. This is sometimes followed by high expectations for academic accomplishments which may not be based on their child's true abilities (McNicol, 1993; Sowell-Coker et al.,1985). Nonetheless, school-related problems represent another significant source of conflict and stress for the West Indian family. Some of the problems they encounter include fighting, poor academic performance, inappropriate placement, discrimination and racism (Clark, 1989; Thomas, 1992; Mahoney, 2002).

Difficulty communicating with school personnel also presents obstacles for West Indian children. For instance, because West Indian Creole is not recognized as a separate language, West Indian children are not eligible to receive the services available to bilingual children. Those who have difficulty making themselves understood are classified as having speech and language disorders. This has resulted in a large number of children who are misclassified and misplaced in special education classes (McNicol, 1993). Communication is also an issue for parents, many of whom have difficulty making their views known to teachers and other school personnel (McNicol, 1993).

NEED FOR A MULTILEVEL APPROACH

The preceding discussion highlights the difficulties facing West Indian families and the need for assistance and support. Given the broad expanse of needs and the complexity of the problems that plague the West Indian family, change efforts must aim not just at the individual and interpersonal levels but should also target those social and economic factors that contribute to the problem.

To accomplish this task, a multilevel approach, which utilizes the micro strategies associated with direct intervention at the individual and interpersonal levels, and the macro strategies of indirect intervention at the institutional and societal levels, is required. This approach stresses the dual responsibility of social workers to both individuals and society. It allows the practitioner to assist individuals with the resolution of a problem while at the same time working for change in the environment. For example, if the goal of intervention is to ensure that children remain in their home, social workers can respond on many levels. On an individual level, they can educate parents about social service laws and provide information to parents on alternative methods for disciplining and controlling children's behavior. For although some parents may see that adaptations must be made, they may be uncertain of how to do this and may have no acceptable role models. On the institutional level, policy changes regarding the criteria for putting children into care may be necessary. Social workers can also advocate for increased funding for family support services and for less emphasis on foster care placement.

Dehoyos et al. (1986) maintain that by moving beyond the level of individuals and their support systems, social workers can be more insightful in their assessment, more effective in problem-solving and more understanding and nonjudgmental. As previously discussed, poor employment opportunities often push West Indian parents into low wage positions that are unstable and usually without health or vacation benefits. As a result, many are forced to take multiple jobs in order to support their families or achieve their goals. However, holding multiple jobs affects their availability to children and makes it difficult for them to make and keep appointments with social service agencies and schools. When this happens some practitioners and school personnel view these parents as neglectful and uncaring. However, it is clear that this problem is not limited to parents but to those social and economic forces that impede their ability to find gainful employment. To deny or to ignore these factors is to ignore the true reality of their external environment.

An orientation which considers both personal and environmental factors aids the practitioner in identifying the unique needs of West Indians and multiple points of intervention in achieving social work goals. This suggests that the worker must undertake intervention strategies which include the concept of advocacy and empowerment.

Advocacy

Sosin and Caulum (1983) define advocacy as an attempt to change the pattern of decision-making on behalf of another who is in a less powerful status than the decision maker. This implies that a power imbalance exists and that the social worker plays an active role in changing those conditions that may impede the mutually beneficial interaction between people and the environment. Social work with West Indians requires advocacy on two levels–on behalf of families to ensure that their interests are being served at the micro level, and policy advocacy in which the worker is an advocate for changes in policy that are conducive to their well-being and development. For example, it requires social workers to advocate for system sensitivity with institutions that lack understanding of this population. As demonstrated earlier, institutions such as the education system are not always sensitive to the needs and challenges faced by immigrant children and their families. In working directly with families social workers can act as a cultural bridge between parents and teachers so that parents are able to make their views known and participate in their children's education. Most parents are also unaware that their children cannot be denied an education because of their immigration status. Social workers can provide information to help parents understand the education system and their rights as parents. Where necessary, they may also need to help parents accept that their children may not be capable of the educational goals which they so much desired.

Empowerment

Influencing the external social system to be more responsive to human needs not only requires advocacy but an empowerment approach that seeks to increase the power and resources of oppressed groups (Pinderhughes, 1983). Empowerment has been defined as "a process whereby persons who belong to a stigmatized social category throughout their lives can be assisted to develop and increase skills in the performance of valued social roles." (Solomon, p. 6). As a strategy in the reduction of powerlessness, empowerment requires the social worker to educate clients about their situation, the power dynamics and the system in which they live, as well as teach them new skills to access resources and act on their own behalf. In this way, they are able to differentiate between those factors in their situation that belong to the external system and those that belong to them (Pinderhuges, 1983). Pierce and Elisme (1997) provide an empowerment practice model for use with oppressed populations that may be useful in working with West Indian families. The model involves three stages: motivation, competence and influence.

The motivation stage is aimed at counteracting powerlessness. For example, because of the reluctance of West Indian families to accept help, Pierce and Elisme (1997) suggest that social workers may need to begin by convincing families of the usefulness of social work services. This may involve providing help with immigration, school related difficulties and other issues that the family saw as particularly problematic or unsolvable. Russell and White (2001) point out that this approach can serve multiple functions including reducing client anxiety, developing trust and establishing a base for discussion of more personal problems.

Competence refers to the ability of immigrant families to control their own lives and involves learning about resources, gaining knowledge, increasing personal and social skills and self assessment (Pierce and Elisme, 1999). Not unlike other immigrant groups, West Indian families are disadvantaged by their lack of understanding of the American system. As such, a necessary task in the empowerment of this population is the provision of information and support to enable them to function in mainstream society. Basic information on how to access food, clothing, housing and so on, is essential. Providing information about employment training programs, the medical, legal and education system is also essential in increasing client competencies.

In the final stage of the model the client is encouraged to use the newly acquired skills and competencies to advocate for permanent change in their community. In the context of the limited support currently provided by government to immigrants, clients can take a leadership role in organizing for community-based services. They can also form coalitions with others to respond to social welfare reform that threatens vulnerable immigrant populations.

CONCLUSION

West Indian families face a complex web of problems in their attempts to integrate into their new society. Some of the challenges they encounter include problems in the parent-child relationship, family role changes, and employment and education-related difficulties. Social work has an important contribution to make in alleviating some of the stresses faced by West Indian families. Its strength lies in the importance it attaches to respect of people, their strengths, customs, and problem-solving capacities. By utilizing a multilevel approach which uses both the micro and macro strategies of social work practice, social work can make a significant contribution in helping individuals and families who are burdened with personal and environmental problems.

REFERENCES

Arnold, E. (1997). Issues in re-unification of migrant West Indian children in the United Kingdom. In J. L. Roopnarine & J. Brown (Eds.), *Caribbean families: Diversity among ethnic groups.* Norwood, NJ: Ablex.

Baker, Frank (1993). "Research shows spanking has long term negative effects." *Children News.*

Baptiste, D., Hardy, K., & Lewis, L. (1997). Clinical practice with Caribbean immigrant families in the United States: The intersection of emigration, immigration, culture and race. In J.L. Roopnarine & J. Brown (Eds.), *Caribbean families: Diversity among ethnic groups* (pp. 275-303). Norwood, NJ: Ablex.

Brice, Janet (1982). "West Indian families." In McGoldrick et al. (Eds.), *Ethnicity and family therapy.* New York, The Guilford Press.

Chau, Kenneth L. (1991). "Social Work with ethnic minorities: Practice issues and potentials."*Journal of Multicultural Social Work,* Vol. 1, 23-39.

Clark, V. (1989). *Perceptions of West Indian parents of their children's placement within the structure and programs of schools in New York City.* New York: Caribbean Research Center, Medgar Evers College.

De Hoyos, Genevieve, De Hoyos, Arturo, & Anderson, Christian B. (1986). "Sociocultural dislocation: Beyond the dual perspective." *Social Work,* Vol. 31, 61-67.

Grasmuck, S., & Grosfoguel, R. (1997). "Geopolitics, economic niches, and gendered social capital among recent Caribbean immigrants in New York City." *Sociological Perspectives,* 40, 339-363.

Kasinitz, P. & Vickerman, M. (2001). "Ethnic niches and racial traps: Jamaicans in the New York regional economy." In Cordero-Guzman, Smith & Grosfoguel (Eds.), *Migration, transnationalization, and race in a changing New York.* Philadelphia: Temple University Press.

Lee, Jik-Jeon, Patcher, Michael A., & Balgopal, Pallassana, R. (1991). "Essential dimensions for developing and delivering services for the Asian American elderly." *Journal of Multicultural Social Work,* Vol. 1, 3-11.

Leo-Rhynie, E. (1997). "Class, race and gendered issues in child rearing in the Caribbean." In J.L. Roopnarine & J. Brown (Eds.), *Caribbean families: Diversity among ethnic groups* (pp. 25-55), Norwood, NJ: Ablex.

Mahoney, Annette M. (2002). "Newly arrived West Indian adolescents: A call for a cohesive social welfare response to their adjustment needs." *Journal of Immigrant and Refugee Services,* Vol. 1, 2002.

Mathews, Lear (1994). "Social Worker's knowledge of client culture and its use in mental health care of English speaking Caribbean immigrants." *Doctoral Dissertation,* Hunter College School of Social Work, City University of New York.

McNicol, Gopaul Sharon-Ann (1993). *Working with West Indian families.* New York: The Guilford Press.

Nulman, Efrem (1983). "Family therapy and advocacy: Directions for the future." *Social Work,* Vol. 28, 19-22.

Padilla, Y. (1997). "Immigrant policy: Issues for social work practice." *Social Work,* Vol. 42, 595-606.

Palmer, R.W. (1995). *Pilgrims from the sun: West Indian migration to America.* New York: Twayne Publishers.

Payne, M. (1989). "Use and abuse of corporal punishment: A Caribbean view." *Child Abuse and Neglect*, Vol. 13, 389-401.

Pierce W., & Erlange Elisme. (1997). "Understanding and working with Haitian families." *Journal of Family Social Work*, Vol. 2, 49-65.

Pinderhughes, Elaine B. (1983). "Empowerment for our clients and for ourselves." *Social Casework*, Vol. 64, 331-38.

Pinderhughes, Elaine (1989). *Understanding race, ethnicity, and power: The key to efficacy in clinical practice*. New York. The Free Press.

Roopnarine, J.L., & Brown, J. (1997). *Caribbean families: Diversity among ethnic groups*. Norwood, NJ: Ablex.

Russell, M., & Bonnie White (2001). "Practice with immigrants and refugees: Social work and client Perspectives." *Journal of Ethnic and Cultural Diversity in Social Work*, Vol. 9, 73-92.

Smith, M.A.B., & Mason, M.A. (1995). "Developmental disability services to Caribbean Americans in New York City." *Journal of Community Practice*, Vol. 2, 87-106.

Solomon, B.M. (1976). *Black empowerment: Social work in oppressed communities*. New York. Columbia University Press.

Sosin, Michael, & Caulum, Sharon (1983). "Advocacy: A conceptualization for social work practice." *Social Work*, Vol. 28, 12-17.

Soto, I.M. (1987). "West Indian child fostering: Its role in migrant exchanges." In Constance R. Sutton & Elsa M. Chaney (Eds.), *Caribbean life in New York City: Sociocultural dimensions*. New York: Center for Migration Studies.

Thomas, T.N. (1992). "Psycho educational adjustment of English speaking Caribbean and Central American immigrant children in the United States." *School Psychology Review*, 21:566-576.

Thrasher, Shirley, & Anderson, Gary (1988). "The West Indian family: Treatment challenges." *Social Casework*, Vol. 69, 171-176.

Impact of the 1996 Welfare Reform and Illegal Immigration Reform and Immigrant Responsibility Acts on Caribbean Immigrants

Velta Clarke

SUMMARY. This paper examines the impact of the 1996 Welfare Reform and Illegal Immigration and Immigrant Responsibility Acts on Caribbean immigrants in the United States. Drawing from the conceptual framework posited by Dye's (1984) *Elite Preference Model* of policy analysis, the author argues that the three laws have created enormous economic and psychological difficulties among families in the United States. Developing countries in the Caribbean region have been severely impacted by the law since they have had to accommodate returning citizens when they are deported under provisions of immigration policies. The question for consideration by this paper is how may the legal and human rights of deportees be balanced against the rights of the U.S. government to secure its borders and ensure the security of its citizens? The paper also addresses issues of immigration, and international relations particularly the north-south dialogue between powerful developed coun-

Velta Clarke, PhD, is Associate Professor of Teacher Education at the State University of New York at Old Westbury (E-mail: Clarkev@oldwestbury.edu).

[Haworth co-indexing entry note]: "Impact of the 1996 Welfare Reform and Illegal Immigration Reform and Immigrant Responsibility Acts on Caribbean Immigrants." Clarke, Velta. Co-published simultaneously in *Journal of Immigrant & Refugee Services* (The Haworth Social Work Practice Press, an imprint of The Haworth Press, Inc.) Vol. 2, No. 3/4, 2004, pp. 147-166; and: *The Health and Well-Being of Caribbean Immigrants in the United States* (ed: Annette M. Mahoney) The Haworth Social Work Practice Press, an imprint of The Haworth Press, Inc., 2004, pp. 147-166. Single or multiple copies of this article are available for a fee from The Haworth Document Delivery Service [1-800-HAWORTH, 9:00 a.m. - 5:00 p.m. (EST). E-mail address: docdelivery@haworthpress.com].

tries such as the United States and small developing states of the Caribbean. *[Article copies available for a fee from The Haworth Document Delivery Service: 1-800-HAWORTH. E-mail address: <docdelivery@haworthpress.com> Website: <http://www.HaworthPress.com> © 2004 by The Haworth Press, Inc. All rights reserved.]*

KEYWORDS. Discriminatory immigration policy, deportation of immigrants, separation of families, health and welfare of immigrants, international relations

INTRODUCTION

In 1996 there occurred an event that was notable, and was to have a serious effect on Caribbean immigrants in the United States and on immigrants in general. The United States Congress overwhelmingly passed three bipartisan bills called the Welfare Reform Act, the Anti-Terrorism Act, and the Illegal Reform and Immigrant Responsibility Act. It was a landmark event. Signed by President Clinton, the Acts were part of the agenda of the Conservative Republican party which had swept into legislative power with the elections of 1994, with an agenda for change. The goals of the Welfare Reform Act were the stimulation of work, the reduction of welfare dependency, and the promotion of family life including healthy marriages and reduction of out-of-wedlock births. The Anti-Terrorism and Immigration Acts were particularly aimed at regulating immigrants, legal residents, undocumented persons as well as refugees.

The paper will focus on the immigrants from the Caribbean, particularly highlighting the impact of the three laws on immigrants and their families. The paper will outline the efforts by Advocacy Organizations, Congress, the Courts, and the Caribbean Community (CARICOM) to seek redress for various forms of injustices resulting from these laws.

POLICY ANALYSIS FRAMEWORK

The decision of the U.S. government to deport immigrants may be described as public policy output and its impact may be analyzed by the methodology of policy analysis. Policy analysis aims at providing explanations of phenomena, and inquires into the context and consequences of policy decisions by using quantitative data, ethnographic information and making inferences.

Through this instrument, the objective observer learns about the policy by studying critical linkages among variables including the social and economic context of the policy initiative, the effects on institutions, and the impact on the target population. The influence of the three laws enacted by the Federal government will be evaluated using the Elite Preference Policy model of policy analysis described thus:

> According to Dye (1984) society is divided into the few who have power and the masses who are powerless. The power elites make decisions about the lives of the masses. Dye suggests that because the elites are generally conservatives, changes in the nature of the system occur when events threaten the social system and elites, acting on the basis of enlightened self-interest, institute reform aimed at preserving the system and their place in it. (p. 29)

Application of the Elite Model

In application of this Model, the elite being considered are those associated with "big business" and members of the U.S. Congress who became the governing party following the mid-term election of 1994. The "earth shattering" matter that threatened the status quo had three aspects: the high incidence of poor citizens on public welfare, immigration, and crime. Welfare recipients, both natives and immigrants, were classified as having the dependency syndrome, relying totally on the "public purse" for support. Their failure to achieve success in the work force was attributed to inherent deficiencies. Poor native citizens and immigrants were targeted as abusers of certain welfare provisions. For example, Borjas (2000) in a study of the use of food stamps argued that immigrant participation in cash benefit programs had risen dramatically since 1970. He argued, further, that it was for this reason that Congress enacted the Welfare Legislation of 1996. The second issue concerns illegal immigration and the third a high incidence of crimes both among those on welfare and among immigrants in general.

The conservative elites were concerned with preserving the American values of limiting the role of government in social welfare provision, promoting self-sufficiency, and social stability. In keeping with conservative values, criminal behavior should be punished harshly with limited emphasis on rehabilitative measures. Conservative values were articulated in the document called "Partnership with America" enunciated by Newt Gingrich, leader of the Congressional House of Representatives. But it was President Clinton, a Democrat, who critics claimed adopted the conservative agenda and signed the bill into law. The Welfare Reform Act and the Illegal Immigration Acts were intended to reduce these disturbing trends of welfare dependency, illegal immigration and crime among the masses, so as to preserve the American system and its values. The Elite Model has four aspects which will be applied to analysis of the Immigration Act. The four prongs are: Analysis of the Economic and Political Context of the Policy; Description of the Policy; The Impact or the Consequences of the Policy on the Target Population; and Institutional Responses to the Consequences.

ECONOMIC, SOCIAL AND POLITICAL CONTEXTS

Immigration occurs in context. Generally, immigration is related to the economy of a country, since most of those who migrate do so because of economic necessity. It is also related to politics since decisions about immigrants who enter a country are made by politicians in order to maintain their power and satisfy their constituents. The acculturation and adjustment of the immigrants within the host country is a socioeconomic process.

Who Are the Immigrants? The International Poor

Most immigrants come to America to seek economic opportunities. Indeed, most Caribbean immigrants are from the unemployed sector of the Caribbean countries, and those from Haiti are classified as both economic and political refugees. Since the 1965 Immigration and Nationality Act, most of those who emigrate from the Caribbean have been the unemployed and the poor. For example, according to INS data, in 1987, 52 percent of the 102,899 legal immigrants from the Caribbean had no occupation, while in 1982 the rate was 59 percent of the 67,379 immigrants. In recent years the data have been reported differently. Data from the Office of Immigration Statistics, Department of Homeland Security for 2001, show that of the 13,634 immigrants from the Caribbean, there were 1,114 visitors, 30 crewmen, 48 students, 58 agricultural workers, 1,119 other workers, 3,093 immigrants, 79 stowaways, 15 in transit without visas, and 8,078 who entered without inspection (p. 13). In effect, most of the immigrants were compromised. Generally, most professionals remain in their own countries, it is the powerless unemployed and those with no occupation who migrate to seek opportunities in the land which states on the Statue of Liberty, *"give me your tired and poor."* These powerless usually arrive with strong work values, expectations for upward mobility, and desire to be valued and respected by their host country.

Rodriquez (1996) in a review of the Act proposed that the international poor workers were being made the "scapegoat." These immigrants from developing countries in Africa, Asia, Latin America and the Caribbean, were anxious for work and were hired by Americans to perform menial tasks abandoned by citizens of this country. According to Rodriquez, those Americans who hire them, constantly degrade them and express impatience with U.S. immigration policies. Census data from the Department of Commerce show that in 1997, 34.7 percent of foreign-born persons had not completed high school, compared with 16 percent of native-born. Also, that 8.4 percent of foreign-born were unemployed compared with 4.3 native-born persons. Further, the poverty rate for naturalized citizens was 10.4 percent, that of foreign-born was 26.8 percent, and that of native-born was 12.9 percent. In effect, foreign-born persons have a significant role but have marginal status in the economy. Despite the major contributions of foreign-born persons to the economic growth of the society, segments of the population express traditional Nativist intolerance towards them and support policies such as the Illegal Immigration and Immigrant Responsibility Act which seeks to deport immigrants for any infringement of the law.

Government's Responsibility to Make Immigration Regulations

Immigration policies are matters dealt with by governments, which have the right to determine the free movement of human beings within their own countries. Governments have the responsibility to regulate their borders, to strengthen the economic and political structures, and to protect and defend its citizenry. Movements among peoples are generally regulated by mutual agreements among sending and receiving countries. That is why the matter of illegal immigrants becomes critical. Some argue that by migrating illegally, immigrants have forfeited their basic human rights, and others contended that governments have a responsibility to uphold human rights whatever the status of the individual. The U.S. Government does not feel compelled to uphold the rights of illegal immigrants who do not generally cooperate with authorities. Moreover, the citizenry complain that by providing cheap labor, illegal immigrants take away jobs from citizens and undermine the economy. Further, many immigrants avail themselves of public benefits such as health services, the school system and welfare provided for citizens, and they become a burden to society. Most of all, some commit crimes. Despite this, unless they are convicted of crimes, the Federal government generally disregards their presence. The media is famous for revealing these inconsistencies in the immigration law.

The Question of Human Rights

According to Kritz and Keeley (1983) the legal conditions under which a person has been granted permission to reside in a particular territory are closely linked to the human and civil rights of the individual. There are in International Law, provisions for rights for all human beings that specifically relate to countries which are signatories to the agreement. For example, labor rights are regulated by the *International Labor Organization* and *Amnesty International* monitors the rights of "criminals." There are also rights which have not been institutionalized and exist only by the goodwill of the individual countries. Countries do not feel obligated to offer rights to non-citizens, who are considered to exist on the periphery or edge of society, and deserve only the *"crumbs"* given by the receiving country. Countries like America have enshrined within its immigration law, expectations that immigrants be self-supporting and not be a burden to society. The United States absolutely does not expect migrant workers to break the law. Theorists like Heurtado (1998) support the government's position. He believes that the most important principle for immigrants is that they all should observe the law, particularly the criminal law, and that any violation should be punished not only by the penalties fixed by the criminal code, but by expulsion from the country. However, there are those who believe that even illegal immigrants have rights such as the right to social assistance that has been enshrined in the behavior of human beings since the dawn of civilization, and was central to the Judeo-Christian tradition which influenced Western Civilization. It is the least that America can do. It must be noted, too, that while illegal immigrants do not have civil rights which are the natural inheritance of Americans, they have human rights which are internationally recognized.

DESCRIPTION OF THE POLICY–THE THREE LAWS

There were three components of the legislation: the Anti-Terrorism and Effective Death Penalty Act signed on April 24, 1996, the Personal Responsibility and Work Reconciliation Act of August 22, 1996 and the Illegal Immigration Reform and Immigration Responsibility Act of September 30, 1996. The Anti-terrorism Act was really directed at immigrants. It was presented to the public as a response to the Oklahoma City bombing of 1995. However, although this fact was little discussed at the time, the purpose of the law was not directly related to terrorism, it was an immigration act (Glaser, 1996). The Act provided for the expedited removal of criminal aliens described as terrorists, use of secret evidence in hearings against non-citizens accused of a crime, and the detention of illegal aliens. It expanded the definition of a crime to include less serious infractions like forgery and perjury (Ma, 1999). The impact was a dramatic increase in the number of incarcerated persons and a complementary increase in the number of prisons, which the government now required private companies to provide. The provision of prisons was good business for the elites in private industry since the drop in the crime rate between 2000 and 2001 had resulted in the loss of business.

THE PERSONAL RESPONSIBILITY AND WORK RECONCILIATION (OR WELFARE REFORM) ACT

The Personal Responsibility and Work Reconciliation Act also called *the Welfare Act (Public Law 104-193)* was signed in August 1996. By the provisions of the Act, benefits for legal immigrants would be cut by 44 percent; it was designed to ensure that available benefits would not serve as an incentive for immigration, and that immigrants to the United States would be self-reliant (Rein, 2022). Legal immigrants, who entered the United States prior to August 1996, would retain eligibility for Supplemental Social Security (SSI) as well as benefits for the aged, blind and disabled. However, the Federal government directed states to bar the pre-reform immigrants from Medicaid, Temporary Assistance to Needy Families (TANF), and food stamps for which they had been previously eligible. Immigrants arriving after August 1996 were summarily barred from all benefits until they became naturalized citizens, when there would be a five-year limit. The ideology of the Personal Responsibility Act was expressed thus in section 2 of the House of Representatives Bill which states, "It continues to be the immigration policy of the United States that,

A. *Aliens within the nation's borders should meet their own needs, should rely on their own capabilities and resources of their families and sponsors and private organizations should not rely on the Federal government for sustenance.*
B. *The availability of public benefits does not constitute an incentive for immigration to the United States, exceptions in case of emergencies."* (Personal Responsibility Act, 1996) 2

Impact of the Welfare Act on Immigrant Families

In implementation, the Welfare Reform Act was fraught with difficulties. It had consequences both on the general American population and on legal and illegal immigrants. The U.S. Accounting Office reported that when the Welfare Reform Act was implemented in 1997, an estimated 940,000 of the 1.4 million legal immigrants receiving food stamps lost their eligibility. In New York City where non-citizens constituted only five percent of the population, they received 40 percent of the cuts. The Office reported that some states had created food stamp programs to serve children, the elderly and disabled who were affected by the Act. By eliminating immediately such benefits as food stamps, and Medicaid for permanent residents, the Act affected the most vulnerable members of the society, the elderly, disabled and children and was deleterious to the family values which it was intended to promote.

For Caribbean immigrants, the Welfare Reform Act had consequences for the pace of citizenship and for poor families. Firstly, there was a dramatic increase in the number of immigrants who became naturalized citizens of the United States. In a study, Singer and Gibertston (2000) found that immigrants from the Dominican Republic were motivated to become citizens, an action which was no doubt driven by the fear of being denied benefits for which they had been entitled prior to the enactment of the law. Secondly, many immigrants were affected by the food stamps policy. George Borjas' (2000) study of the use of food stamps by immigrants showed that immigrants of the lower socioeconomic status depended on food stamps. Hence the Welfare Reform Act which eliminated assistance to them was particularly difficult for their families. However, Fremstad (2000) in his study showed that Caribbean immigrants were mindful of the provision that they should not become "a public charge." Further, many West Indians stayed away from Welfare benefits for two reasons: (1) Illegal immigrants could not risk becoming entangled with the INS and (2) Some legal immigrants were too proud to seek welfare as they were constrained by their West Indian cultural values, which frowned upon dependence on public assistance.

Institutional Response to the Welfare Law

American social and political institutions including the Congress and the Courts are politically conscious groups which understand the powers of negative public opinion and negative perceptions, and they understood that a dissatisfied public could destabilize their power. Accordingly, they made prompt responses to the Welfare Law. By a series of Acts, Congress addressed some of the injustices in the Welfare law. In 1997, the Balanced Budget Act (PL 105-34) restored Social Security Income (SSI) and Medicaid benefits to legal immigrants who had received them prior to the passage of the welfare law. In June 1998, the Agricultural Research and Extension and Education Reform Act (PL 105-185) restored food stamps to the same group and in October 1998, the Non-Citizen Benefit Clarification and Other Technical Amendment Act (PL 105-306) restored SSI and Medicaid benefits. In all, by November 1998 eligible immigrants who had received benefits before the enactment of the welfare legislation, children, persons over 65 years old, and the disabled, recovered benefits of food stamps, SSI and Medicaid.

According to Rein (2003), the groups of beneficiaries comprised 250,000 immigrants. Further, according to the Legislative Update (1999), Senator Daniel Moynihan and Representative Sander Levin in 1999 sponsored the Fairness for Legislation Act which permitted States to give Medicaid coverage to children, restore food stamp benefits to victims of domestic violence, and to all qualified immigrants who had lived in the U.S. before 1996. A bill by John Chafee legislated benefits to immigrant children and pregnant women.

THE ILLEGAL IMMIGRATION REFORM AND IMMIGRANT RESPONSIBILITY ACT (IIRIRA)

The Illegal Immigration Reform and Immigrant Responsibility Act signed on September 30, 1996, had the following provisions:

The law gave sweeping powers to the Immigration and Naturalization Service to determine admissions, deportation and detention of immigrants who had committed crimes. Legal residents could be deported, and those who were seeking asylum could be denied even humanitarian aid (House of Representatives Act 3734, 1996).

The Act toughened penalties for immigrants convicted of smuggling, increased detention space for criminals, and instituted and expedited removal or denial of a hearing of criminals convicted of a felony. It required that all legal immigrants convicted of a crime be confined and deported without the possibility of relief. It further expanded the definition of crime to mean "*aggravated felony*" which in effect meant minor crimes such as drug offenses, shoplifting or check kiting for which a sentence of one year was imposed by a judge. Other legal immigrants who committed petty thefts or burglary had to be deported even if they were sentenced for a year and had never served a day in jail. In addition, legal immigrants who had lived in the U.S. for years could be deported for misdemeanors even without a prison term.

Moreover, aggravated felony was retroactive, so that crimes committed years ago and for which the person had already served time, was released from prison, and was now living an exemplary life, was punishable by deportation.

Furthermore, immigrants had no rights to habeas corpus or judicial review by a federal court. The Act restricted the power of the federal courts to review any individual deportation or to issue injunctions against INS policies even though that agency was acting illegally. In effect, the Act was an attack on the authority of the court and the rule of law, and represented discrimination against immigrants.

Lastly, the Act required an affidavit of 125 percent of income above the poverty level for an individual who sponsored immigrants. Sponsors had to have resources of at least $17,761 income for a family of four, and an income of $24,636 for a family of six.

Impact of the Act on Immigrants

The impact of the Act was dramatic on immigrants, refugees and those on welfare. It increased significantly the number of immigrants incarcerated. White (2002) reported that since the 1996 the number of immigrants detained tripled from 5,532 to 19,533. These were persons seeking asylum, waiting to be deported or charged with a crime. In addition, the number of offenders serving sentences rose from 18,929 to 35, 629. Jason Ma (1999) of the *Asian Week* reported that between October 1998 and June 1999, 47,000 persons were deported and of these 47 percent had been convicted of drug-related crimes and 14 percent for violent crimes.

Immigrants Detained in Jails

When the law was enacted there were not enough detention facilities to accommodate offenders, thus Congress delayed the mandatory detention until 1998. However, the INS in its zealous, anti-immigrant fervor, became very aggressive and detained prisoners in county jails, federal prisons, and private lockups. Aliens without a criminal record and those seeking asylum were held in the toughest jails. *The Dallas Morning News* of April 1, 2001 under the Freedom of Information Act found that 851 persons from 69 countries were held without due process for at least three years, including 60 felons and 360 innocent persons.

Deportees to the Caribbean Region

Table 1 shows that between 1997 and 2002, a total of 38,614 Caribbean immigrants of English, French, Spanish and Dutch descents, including both criminals and non-criminals, were deported. Crimes for which immigrants have been deported include: burglary, domestic violence, driving with suspended licenses, possession of guns and drugs, murder, rape and sexual abuse of children. The numbers compiled from Tables 46 and 48 of the yearbook are shown in Table 1.

In addition to those deported, the data show that another group of immigrants from the Caribbean were under "*docket control*" and earmarked to de-

TABLE 1

	Criminal	Non-Criminal	Total
Caribbean Region	**25,716**	**12,898**	**38,614**
Anguilla	6	8	14
Antigua-Barbuda	166	54	220
Aruba	16	12	28
The Bahamas	479	104	537
British Virgin Island	18	8	26
Cayman Island	6	4	10
Cuba	371	60	431
Dominica	207	51	258
Dominican Republic	12,415	6,851	19,266
Grenada	100	47	147
Haiti	1,897	954	2,857
Jamaica	8,000	3,749	11,749
Martinique	6	9	15
Montserrat	1	0	11
St. Kitts	107	15	122
St. Lucia	107	51	158
St. Vincent	109	61	170
Trinidad and Tobago	1,151	776	1,927
Turks and Caicos Islands	19	8	27
TOTALS	25,355	12,898	38,614

Source: Immigration and Naturalization Service Yearbook, 1997-2002.

part based on their criminal status. The numbers including both criminals and non-criminals were 573 in 2000, 576 in 2001 and 432 in 2002.

Data from the U.S. Sentencing Commission showed that generally these defendants tended to be younger, and less well-educated. Of those sentenced, 51 percent were non-citizens and 42 percent citizens of the United States. Also, of those citizens sentenced, 60 percent were high school graduates, and comparatively, 30 percent of non-citizens were high school graduates.

Families Separated and Impoverished

The deportation of immigrants has been found to have a deleterious effect on families. When the breadwinner, usually the male, is deported, families are often left without visible means of support. Many of those family members have had to seek available pubic assistance. It is particularly difficult for pregnant women and children. The irony is that the welfare reforms purported to promote unified families, and so deportation of the head of the household was inimical to the family values that the law was intended to promote. Further, the wealth, health, and well-being of families were further affected by the fragmentation of families. Ku and Blaney (2000) of the Center of Budget and Policy Priorities analyzed the Census data describing the health insurance coverage of immigrant children and deduced that the health of low-income children and their parents had become more precarious since the passage of the law of 1996, as many of these families had lost insurance coverage. Generally, when a breadwinner loses his job, he is also deprived of health benefits.

Deportation and Mental Health

The U.S deportation policy has had a devastating effect on the social welfare of Caribbean countries as well as the mental health of the deportees themselves, in ways that have raised serious questions about the justice of the law. *The Jamaican Daily Gleaner* of November 19, 2003 commented on the implementation of the law thus, "within the last seven years 17,000 persons were deported to Jamaica alone and of these, 12,000 were listed as being engaged in criminal activity. In essence, one in every 106 young men in Jamaica is a criminal deportee from the United States."

The plight of deportees was discussed at the 12th Annual Conference of the Faculty of Medicine of the University of the West Indies. *The Jamaican Daily Gleaner* reported on a study conducted by a group of researchers led by Drs. Freddie Hickling and Wendell Holmes of the University. They had studied 15 deportees from the United States and found that most of them were suffering from "schizophrenia, bipolar disorder and substance abuse." The deportees were respectable, college-educated men some of whom were veterans of the U.S. army. The report highlighted the case of a 42-year-old man who had left Jamaica at the age of 13. He served in the U.S. army, had no criminal history, and was later discharged from service when he was diagnosed with schizophrenia. The article goes on to say that he had assaulted a staff member and for this crime he was deported. The man had no family in Jamaica, little knowledge of the country of his birth and because of illness had no means of supporting himself. When the United States authorities deported him, they had full knowledge of his exemplary service, his lack of criminal background, the absence of family connections in Jamaica, his poor financial status, and his illness. Under the circumstances, his deportation could be regarded as an inconsiderate act. The experiences of other mentally ill veterans with a history of criminal behavior who had been deported under the provisions of the Illegal Immigrant Act. In fact, the conference on mental health was convened to discuss the plight of the deported mentally ill persons, and discuss the policy implications for addressing their needs. These cases highlight the human suffering emanating from this Act.

Increase in Criminal Activity in Caribbean Countries

The data in Table 1 show that since the Illegal Immigrant Law was enacted, thousands of immigrants from the Caribbean region have been deported. The repatriation of deportees has been very difficult for Caribbean nations. Some of those deported were already criminals in the United States. Further, the immigration data show that most of them had no skills and on returning to the Caribbean their hopes of acquiring a skill were even more remote. Their option for survival has been to commit more crimes. It has been shown that several criminal actions in the Caribbean region were committed by *deportees* from America.

Institutional Responses to the Immigration Law

The United States government and various organizations have responded to the problems caused by the immigration acts. Like the Welfare Reform Act, American social and political institutions including Advocacy organizations, the Federal Government, the Congress, and the Courts were constrained to make changes to the laws in order to redress injustice, minimize the suffering of the target population, and avoid the wrath of citizens and consequent political impact. Voluntary organizations have had a critical role in advocating for change to the immigration law. Asian organizations including the National Asian Pacific American Legal Consortium, Asian Pacific American Legal Center, Northern California Coalition for Immigrants have joined in a campaign to "*Fix 96.*"

Another organization which has been concerned with the plight of immigrants is the Congress for Racial Equality (CORE). CORE's main concern is with immigrants from Africa and the Caribbean and their basic civil and human rights. Immigrants from the English-speaking Caribbean have advocates in their governments through the organization called Caribbean Community (CARICOM). The general hostility to the Act led to a march on Washington in October 1996, when Congresswoman Nydia Velazquez of New York City and tens of thousands of Latinos marched against what was perceived as an anti-immigrant and anti-Latino Policy. Congress has also addressed the issue of deportation of immigrants.

To redress these apparently inhumane results, Congress introduced a bipartisan Family Reunification Act of 1999. Introduced by Representatives Frank and Frost, it proposed a limit on the types of crimes for which legal immigrants could be deported, put limitations on the mandatory detention provision making it possible for felons who were not threats to the community to be released, and restored to these immigrants, the right to appeal. Before 1996, immigrants convicted of a crime could be released on parole after six months of imprisonment and were allowed to remain in the U.S. However, under the 1996 law, the INS could detain criminals indefinitely even after they had completed their prison term. This issue was contested in the cases of *Zadvydas vs. Davis* and *Ashcroft v. Ma*. In a majority decision (5-4), the U.S. Supreme Court ruled that the 1996 law could not be applied retroactively to crimes committed before 1996 and that all immigrants facing deportation should have the right to judicial review. The court ruled that the government could not detain deportable aliens just because their home countries would not accept them and that the government should have a special reason for keeping in custody immigrants who had already served a prison term for a crime. In effect, the Court clarified that the Federal government had to be subject to the Constitution including the right to due process.

In July 2001, Attorney General John Ashcroft directed the INS to release 3,400 prisoners who had completed prison terms and whose countries had refused to take them back. These immigrants who were called *"lifer"* numbered about 1,000 of the 3,400 detainees. Among them were several hundreds from Jamaica who had refused to be repatriated, claiming that it was their lives in the United States which has made them hardened criminals. The Attorney General promised to take strong action against countries that resisted or delayed taking back their nationals. He would refuse to issue visas to these countries.

Response of the Federal Administration

According to Best (2002), the Bush Administration has reaffirmed its commitment to uphold the 1996 Immigration law and has argued against the provision of funds for the repatriation of immigrant deportees who have been convicted of crimes in the United States. The position was made clear by the U.S. Immigration and Naturalization Service (INS), now part of U.S. Department of Citizenship and Homeland Security. Secondly, the Administration was firm that there were no plans to change the U.S. laws to facilitate the breadwinners of families. The Administration gave little hope that there would be imminent changes in the Immigration law that should make it possible to help families. Although there were bills pending in Congress, the response of the Administration was that *these bills were very much a work in progress and there was no guarantee that the 107th Congress which was ending would enact them into law*.

Advocacy of CARICOM

The matter of the implications of the Welfare Law and immigration laws was discussed in 2002, at a meeting of the Caribbean Community (CARICOM) at which U.S. Secretary of State Colin Powell was present. CARICIOM Ministers asked that seized assets be used to help Caribbean countries and further to take into account the "disruptive effect repatriation had on families in the native countries." The countries of the region asked the Bush administration for:

- financial help for repatriation of these deportees
- financial help for those whose families had lost the wage earner
- a halt in the number of persons being deported and an end to mandatory deportation

The Bush administration made it clear that forfeited assets could not be used for deported convicts or their families. The best offer by the Justice Department was to offer "technical assistance and training programs" to help countries in devising forfeiture legislation. CARICOM countries could submit a proposal to the respective embassies and the U.S. administration would consider giving assistance for "parole and for the monitoring" of convicts. Thirdly, the Bush administration refused to consider an end to mandatory deportations, pointing out that *"all nations have an obligation to take back their nationals."*

IMPLICATIONS FOR U.S. IMMIGRATION POLICY

The question of immigration both legal and illegal has strong implications for U.S. foreign policy and international relations. In the North-South dialogue, legal immigration is not discussed as a social or legal phenomenon, but only in economic terms as a brain drain, or in terms of the transfer of labor and technology. Also, the questions of illegal immigration, and the social, political and legal issues they pose are generally ignored. However, immigration raises issues of human rights and treatment of immigrants, which are generally ignored.

Immigrants and Human Justice

Some of the provisions of The Illegal Immigration Reform and Immigrant Responsibility Act may be viewed as discriminatory and antithetical to basic human justice. The proposal that legal residents who had paid taxes and contributed to the economy should be punished twice for a crime may be considered as an injustice. Caribbean immigrants have shown a determination to challenge the laws concerning deportation and have adopted the defense of family hardship which was the basis of the original law. In this regard two immigrants from the Caribbean have successfully defended their claims and won resounding reversals based on family hardships. In the case of *Calcano-Martinez v. INS* September 2001, Deboris Calcano-Martinez of the Dominican Republic was admitted to the U.S in 1971 at the age of three as a permanent resident. A mother of four, she was in 1997 found guilty of heroin possession, and earmarked for deportation. When she appealed to the Second Circuit of Appeals for habeas corpus review, she won the right to have her case reviewed based on family reunification principles and on constitutional grounds that the federal court can review the claims of an alien against deportation.

The second case was that of Enrico St. Cyr, a Haitian resident lawfully admitted to the U.S. in 1986, and convicted of drug trafficking in 1996. His conviction was based on the Anti-Terrorism and Effective Death Penalty Act and the Illegal Immigration Reform and Immigrant Responsibility Act. In 1999, he appealed against deportation to the District of Connecticut Court on the basis that the law was being applied retroactively and that deportation would cause extreme family hardship. In 1999 the Court ruled in his favor, that the law may not be applied to an alien if the crime, the proceedings and conviction occurred prior to the 1996 legislation.

There is an interplay of four factors in these two cases: they were both legal permanent residents, they both possessed drugs, the law was applied retroactively and the appeal was made on the basis of extreme family hardship. It can also be agreed that citizens who break U.S. law should be punished but due process should be applied in accordance with the Fourteenth Amendment of the American Constitution. Thus the U.S. should not make punishment by deportation retroactive for those who had committed crimes in the past, and had already served their time for which they were convicted. This is double jeopardy and is contrary to American jurisprudence. *The Courts have set boundaries for deportation of legal immigrants and this has set a precedent for future action.* Generally, when the immigrant who breaks the law is deported he or she leaves the family behind in the U.S. and also a whole sequence of economic consequences and social harm. The deportees have no homes in the native land, and since homelessness is relatively unknown in the Caribbean countries, a new problem is exported to the region. There are also psychological harm and mental illness experienced by the deportees as evidenced by the case of the 42-year-old man described above. Most deportees are legal U.S. citizens who have paid taxes, and made contributions to this country. Accordingly, under the U.S. Constitution, they have inalienable civil rights, and as a corollary, this country has a social responsibility to them. Hence the U.S. should not export them, and the attendant problems to the Caribbean.

Immigration Policy

The United States can again monitor its borders if it resolves the political and economic issues, as well as issues of special interests. Generally, entrepreneurs want immigrants, legal or illegal, for the cheap labor they provide, and politicians want their votes. When the United States resolves these critical issues, then it will be able to take firm steps to regulate immigration. The defensible policy will be to sift incoming immigrants, not on the basis of race as in the past, but on the basis of the needs of the economy for skilled personnel. In 1990 the U.S enacted the Immigration Reform and Control Act (IMMACT) which was directed to skilled workers. It was called a diversity program but was directed to Europeans and also repealed the ban on persons from communist nations. It also admitted immigrants from countries suffering natural disasters.

Accordingly, the U.S. needs a similar policy for countries from the Caribbean. Caribbean countries need their most skilled persons for development. Such a policy should be directed at those persons with potential for providing skills. In this regard the U.S. should *require that those who enter the country without skills, have a plan to obtain a skill suitable for employment as a precondition for entry.* Persons who can provide for themselves are less likely to engage in unlawful economic activities. By carefully selecting immigrants the U.S. will ensure that only persons with the most suitable qualifications, the highest integrity, *and the greatest motivation to acquire skills and provide for themselves enter the country.* Respectable and hardworking persons are less likely to violate the law, will not become a burden on the country, and will promote the highest level of contribution to the United States. It is then and only then that the problems of immigration, and the resulting issues of deportation of criminals, the separation of families, and repatriation of children of permanent residents, and of legal residents who commit crimes, will be alleviated.

CONCLUSION FOR INTERNATIONAL RELATIONS

The 1996 welfare and immigration legislations have had far-reaching impact on a significant number of immigrants. There have been implications for Caribbean immigrants including the impact on the native countries, matters of human justice and civil rights.

The matter of deportation of immigrants is accorded little attention and appears to be of little concern to politicians in developed countries. It is the international poor countries whose citizens commit crime that have a problem. It is a critical problem since deported citizens impose a cost for repatriation and more importantly they take criminal behavior back to the developing country and raise the level of criminal activity in these countries. It is generally agreed that anyone who breaks the law should be punished, but punishment should be done with justice, not with elitist attitudes of retribution. Many immigrants who committed crimes were born in the U.S. and had never been in the country of their parents' birth, having learned their behavior in this country. Deportation of such persons places undue pressure on the economy, security institutions, social services, and health care facilities of the receiving countries. The disruption to family life, the nucleus of a stable society, is extremely critical since developing countries have no experiences with problems like homelessness and social welfare. The U.S. should not deport persons with mental illness nor persons who are U.S. citizens and except in extreme circumstances, should deal with them in accordance with U.S. laws. This country should rationalize aspects of the law that concern families and the deportation of criminals who were born of foreign immigrants in this country.

The 2000 Census data show that 28.4 million residents of the U.S. are foreign born and that they are mostly from Asia, Latin America and the Caribbean, in fact they are people of color. Of the foreign-born, Lisa Lollack shows that 34.5 percent are from Latin America, 15.3 percent from Europe, 25.5 percent from Asia, 6.6 percent from South America, 8.1 percent from other regions and a significant 6.6 percent from the Caribbean. The implications are that these residents have sufficient voting power to influence U.S. policy concerning immigration. Indeed, according to Quiroz-Martinez (2001), because of the 1965 Immigration Act which changed the color and race of immigration, many organizations have been formed to defend the rights of immigrants, and Simmons (2001) suggests that there needs to be some specific antiracist goals. There is also the CARICOM whose constituency is the English-speaking Caribbeans. The power of immigrants may be seen in California where they cooperate as a critical voting block in a number of election districts as in 1997 when they helped to defeat Republican Congressman Dornan, a leading opponent of immigrant rights. As an increasing number of immigrants become citizens, they will increase their power and politicians will be unable to disregard their needs. In the United States there are 3,525,703 Caribbean immigrants who constitute nine percent of the foreign-born American population and their descendants. They should be able to influence U.S. policy concerning the rights of immigrants accordingly.

By deporting immigrants, and disrupting their lives and that of their families, the Illegal Immigration Reform and Immigrant Responsibility Act has demonstrated the effectiveness of the *Elite Model* of policy-making. The impact of the Act has also shown that under pressure, policymakers will make adjustments to an unjust and unpopular policy decision. In effect, these outcomes suggest that immigrants may seek their human and civil rights through the political process and use the power of their numbers to effect changes in immigration policy. Because of their significant numbers and their strategic significance to the U.S. economy, Caribbean immigrants, organizations and governments have enough power to influence the international governments to place issues of immigration and the rights of immigrants on the international agenda as part of the north-south dialogue. It also suggests that immigrants have responsibilities to the host country, the United States, to obey the laws of the land and contribute to its economic development.

REFERENCES

Barone, Michael (2000). Changing Minds, in *U.S. News and World Report*, Vol. 131, Issue 4, p. 25.

Best, Tony (2002). "Voices must be Heard." in *Carib News*, New York, December 10, p. 3.

Borjas George (2000). "Immigration and the Food Stamp Program," Center for Investment Policy, Denver, CO. *jcpr.org/wp/Wprofile.cfm?Id-130*

Dye, Thomas (1984). *Understanding Public Policy*, Englewood, N.J: Prentice Hall, p. 29.

Fremstad, Shawn (2000). What it Means for Immigrants Who Need Public Assistance, Washington, DC: *Center on Budget and Policy Priorities*, p. 7.

Glaser, Ira (1996). "Scapegoating Immigrants-Again," in *Visions of Liberty*, November, 1996, p. 5.

Heurtado, Jesus (1998). A Liberation Theory of Free Immigration, in *Journal of Liberation Studies, 13.2*.

House of Representative Act 3734 (1996). Personal Responsibility and Work Opportunity Reconciliation Act, Section 400, page 2. *http://thomas.loc.gov*

Jamaican Daily Gleaner, November 19, 2003.

Kritz, Mary, Keeley, Charles, & Tomasi, Silvano (Eds.) (1983). *Global Trends in Migration*. New York: Center for Migration Studies.

Ku, Leighton & Blaney, Shannon (2002). "Health Coverage for Legal Immigrant Children, *Center on Budget and Policy Priorities*, p. 10.

Ma, Jason (1999). "Groups Join to Restore immigrants' Rights" in *Asian Week*, Thursday, September 2. p. 4.

"Mentally Ill Deportees" presented at the 12th Annual Conference of the Faculty of Medicine of the University of the West Indies. Published by the *Jamaican Daily Gleaner*, November 19, 2003, p. 19.

Migration News (2001). "U.S Supreme Court Eases 96 Laws" in *Migration News*, Volume 8, Number 8, p. 5.

Morse, Jodie (2002). "A Bleak Verdict on Welfare Reform" in *Time Canada*, Vol. 15, Issue 16, p. 12.

NAKASEC (1999). *Legislative Update*, National Korean American Service and Education Consortium, August, 1999, p. 4.

Quiroz-Martinez (2001). Missing Link, Race Across Borders, *Color Line, Vol. 4, No. 2*. Summer, p. 1.

Rein Mei Ling (2002). *Immigration and Illegal Aliens: Burden or Blessing*, New York: Gale Group.

Rodriquez, R. (1996). Welfare Reform Scapegoats the Easy Target, in *Pacific News Service*, San Francisco, CA. Page, 2.16.

Simmons, (2001). Quoted In: *Missing Link, Race Across Borders, ColorLines*, Vol. 4, No. 2, Summer 2001 p. 1.

Singer, Audrey, & Gilberston, Greta (2000). Naturalization in the Wake of Anti-Immigrant Legislation: The Case of Dominican Immigrants in New York City, in: *International Migration Program, page 5*.

U.S. Department of Citizenship and Homeland Security, Office of Immigration Statistics (2003). *Deportable Aliens by Region and Country of Nationality*, Government Printing Office, p. 13.

White, Roger (2002). "Criminalizing Immigrants," in: *The Fortune Society News*. Winter, 2002 p. 2.

Index

Acculturation
of Caribbean immigrants
of Caribbean women
immigrants, 93-97
post-September 11, 2001, 78-79
definition of, 93
Acquired immunodeficiency syndrome
(AIDS). *See* HIV/AIDS
Adolescents
Caribbean-American, dating
violence among, 103-116
cultural factors in, 105-107
differentiated from adult
domestic violence, 105
school-based prevention model
for, 107-115
gender identity development in, 105
West Indian, migration-related
stress in, 139
Advocacy, 141,142
Africa
HIV/AIDS prevalence in, 50
HIV/AIDS-related mortality rate in,
51
African Americans, infant mortality
rate among, 31
African-American women, heart
disease among, 31
Aging policy, implications for older
West Indian immigrant
women, 25,26
Agricultural Research and Extension
and Education Reform Act of
1998, 154
AIDS. *See* HIV/AIDS
American Apartheid (Massey and
Denton), 4-5
Amnesty International, 152

Anti-Terrorism and Effective Death
Penalty Act of 1996, 162
Elite Preference Policy Analysis of,
152-153
immigrants as targets of, 152-153
Ashcroft, John, 160
Ashcroft v. *Ma,* 160
Asian Pacific American Legal Center,
159
Asian Week, 156
Australia, infant mortality rate in, 31

Bahamas, HIV/AIDS prevalence in,
54,55
Balanced Budget Act of 1997, 154
Barbadian immigrants, in New York
City, 3
Barbados
domestic violence in, 119-130
Domestic Violence Act
(restraining orders) and,
119-120,122,125-130
magistrates' rulings regarding,
128-129
police responses to,
126,127-128,130
societal indifference toward,
119-120
women's power of agency and,
126-131
economy of, 121,122
HIV/AIDS prevalence in, gender
factors in, 57
legal system of, 122
marriage and divorce rate in, 122
women's social status in, 121-122
Beckles, Penelope, 124

Bedford Stuyvesant Community
    Mental Heath Center, 74
Belgium, infant mortality rate in, 31
Belize, HIV/AIDS prevalence in, 55
"Black Success" model, 18,25
British immigrants, infant mortality
    rate among, 40
Brooklyn, New York
    Bedford Stuyvesant Community
        Mental Heath Center, 74
    Crown Heights, HIV/AIDS cases
        in, 59
    residential segregation in, 4-5
Bush Administration, 160,161

Calcano-Martinez, Debaris, 162
Calcano-Martinez v. INS, 162
Canada, infant mortality rate in, 31
CAREC (Caribbean Epidemiology
    Centre), 54,55
Caribbean Community (CARICOM),
    159,161
Caribbean Epidemiology Centre
    (CAREC), 54,55
Caribbean immigrants. See also West
    Indian immigrants
    deportation of, for criminal
        behavior, 155-163
    Bush Administration's response
        to, 160,161
    impact on deported immigrants,
        156,158-159,162
    impact on families of
        immigrants, 157-158
    international relations aspect of,
        163-164
    mental health effects of,
        158-159,162
    economic importance of, 2,3
    effect of welfare reform on, 154
    illegal, 150
    in New York City, 84
    poverty of, 150-151
    psychological disorders in, 4

racism toward, 4,5
remittances to families by, 3,72
social mobility of, 3-4
unemployed status of, 150
as World Trade Center terrorist
    attack victims, 70-71
Caribbean people, definition of, 2
Caribbean region. See also specific
    Caribbean countries
    HIV/AIDS in, 50,54-56
    gender factors in, 56-58
    U.S. immigration policy toward,
        163
Caribbean women, HIV/AIDS among,
    56-58
    role of poverty in, 57-58
Caribbean women immigrants. See
    also West Indian older
    women immigrants
    acculturation of, 93-97
    child fostering practices of, 85
    as "live-in" domestic servants,
        84-85
    migration-related decision-making
        processes in, 83-101
        during acculturation, 93-97
        active planning process, 89
        active preparation process, 91
        conscious awareness process,
            88-89
        critical thinking process, 90-91
        grief, 88-89,97,98
        internal struggling, 95-97
        during migration, 91-93
        prior to migration, 87-91
        relief and hope, 94-95
        resolve, 97
        subconscious awareness process,
            87,88
        support network development,
            85,89-90,96,97
    in New York City, 84
Caribbean Women's Health
    Association, 64

CARICOM (Caribbean Community),
159,161,164
Centers for Disease Control and
Prevention (CDC), 61
Chafee, John, 155
Child abuse, by West Indian parents,
138
Child fostering
among West Indian immigrants,
138-139
definition of, 85
immigrant women's decision
making about
during acculturation, 93-97
during migration, 91-93
prior to migration, 88-91
as transnational mothering, 95-96
Child prostitutes, HIV/AIDS in, 58
Child protective services, 136
Chlamydia infections, 59
Church of England, 121
Clinton, Bill, 148,149
Communication problems, of West
Indian and Caribbean
immigrants, 37,40-41,44,140
Community involvement model, of
HIV/AIDS prevention,
53-54,64-65
Community Needs Index (CNI), 59
Community services and benefits. *See*
Social services and benefits
Condoms, 56,61,62-63
Congress for Racial Equality (CORE),
159
Corporal punishment, West Indian
parents' use of, 137,138
Creole, West Indian, 140
Crime rate, among immigrants, 149
Criminal behavior, of immigrants, 151
as basis for deportation, 155-161
Bush Administration's response
to, 160,161
Elite Preference Policy Analysis
of, 148-150

impact on deported immigrants,
156,158-159,162
impact on families of
immigrants, 157-158
implication for international
relations, 163-164
mental health effects of,
158-159,162
Criminals, human rights of, 152
Critical incident stress, 73
Crown Heights, Brooklyn, HIV/AIDS
cases in, 59

Dallas Morning News, 156
Dating violence, among
Caribbean-American
adolescents, 103-116
cultural factors in, 105-107
differentiated from adult domestic
violence, 105
school-based prevention model for,
107-115
intervention group component
of, 111-112
parent/community awareness
component of, 111
school staff awareness
component of, 110-111
student awareness component of,
109-110
young men's early intervention
group component of, 112-114
young women's early
intervention group
component of, 114-115
Deportation, of Caribbean immigrants
after September 11, 2001,
72,75,76,78
for criminal behavior, 155-161
Bush Administration's response
to, 160,161
Elite Preference Policy Analysis
of, 148-150

impact on deported immigrants,
    156,158-159,162
impact on families of
    immigrants, 157-158
implication for international
    relations, 163-165
mental health effects of,
    158-159,162
Detention, of Caribbean immigrants,
    156. *See also* Prisons
after September 11, 2001, 72,78
Discipline, West Indian parents' style
    of, 137-138
Discrimination
    toward Caribbean immigrants,
        94,106
    after September 11, 2001,
        71-72,75
    toward HIV-infected persons,
        62,63-64
Domestic violence, in Caribbean
    communities, 117-134
    in Barbados, 119-130
        Domestic Violence Act
            (restraining orders) and,
            119-120,122,125-130
        magistrates' rulings regarding,
            128-129
        police responses to,
            126,127-128,130
        societal indifference toward,
            119-120
        women's power of agency and,
            126-131
    implication of immigration policy
        for, 130-132
    restraining orders and, 118,119
        in Barbados,
            119-120,122,125-130
    victims of
        children of, 118
        learned helplessness in, 120
        shelters for, 119
        victims' power of agency and,
            120-121

Dominican Republic
    HIV/AIDS prevalence in, 54
    in child prostitutes, 58
    gender factors in, 57
    immigrants from, as naturalized
        citizens, 154
Dornan, Robert, 164
Dual citizenship, 85

East Indians, discrimination towards,
    71,76
Educational level, of immigrants, 151
Elderly Caribbean immigrants, 5-6.
    See also West Indian older
        women immigrants
    psychological reactions to
        September 11, 2001, 75-76
Elite Preference Policy Analysis,
    148-150
    of Anti-Terrorism and Effective
        Death Penalty Act of 1996,
        152-153
    of Illegal Immigration Reform and
        Immigrant Responsibility Act
        of 1996, 149-150,151,152,
        155-161,163,165
    of Personal Responsibility and
        Work Reconciliation Act of
        1996, 152,153-155
Employment status
    of undocumented women
        immigrants, 85
    of West Indian immigrants
        social services interventions for,
            141
        as source of family
            conflict/stress, 139-140,141
Empowerment, of West Indian
    immigrant families,
    141,142-143
English-language usage, among West
    Indian and Caribbean
    immigrants, 37,40-41,44,140
Ethnic minority elders. *See also*
    Elderly Caribbean

immigrants; West Indian
   older women immigrants
   underutilization of community
   services by, 12
European Americans, as percentage of
   total U.S. population, 12
Extended family, of West Indian
   immigrants, 137,138

Family conflict/stress issues, affecting
   West Indian and Caribbean
   immigrants, 136-140
   child rearing practices, 137-138
   employment, 139-140,141
   family relationships, 137
   parent-adolescent relationship,
      106-107
   parent-child separation and
      reunification (child
      fostering), 138-139
   during acculturation, 93-97
   during migration, 91-93
   prior to migration, 88-91
   school-related problems, 140
Family Reunification Act of 1999,
   159-160
Family structure, of West Indian
   immigrants, 137
Female-headed households
   in the Caribbean region, 57
   in Jamaica, 137
Food stamps, immigrants' eligibility
   for, 149,153-154,155
Freedom of Information Act, 156

Gender identity, development of, 105
Gender relations, in Caribbean
   populations. *See also*
   Domestic violence
   implication for HIV/AIDS
      transmission, 56-57
Gender roles

culturally-defined, 106-107
   socialization into, 105
   of West Indian women and men,
      137
Gerontology, "male worker model" of,
   14
Ghanian immigrants, infant mortality
   rate among, 40
Gingrich, Newt, 149
Globalization, 85-86
Gonorrhea, 59
Grenada, annual migration from, 2
Grenadines, HIV/AIDS-related deaths
   in, 55
Guyana
   annual migration from, 3
   deportation negotiations with the
      United States, 78
   HIV/AIDS among pregnant women
      in, 57
Guyanese immigrants
   infant mortality rate among, 40
   in New York City, 3

Haiti, HIV/AIDS prevalence in, 54,55
   gender factors in, 57
Haitian immigrants
   as economic and political refugees,
      150
   infant mortality rate among, 39,40
Haitian migrant workers, HIV/AIDS
      prevalence among, 61
Hartford, Connecticut, study of older
      West Indian women
      immigrants in, 11-28
Health insurance coverage, for
      immigrants, 158
Health Keepers Model, 44
Healthy People 2000, 31,32
Healthy People 2010, 31
Heart disease, among
      African-American women,
      31

Help-seeking behavior, of Caribbean
    immigrants, 79
Hickling, Freddie, 158
HIV/AIDS, 49-67
    among homosexuals,
        51,55,59-60,61-62
    attitudes toward HIV/AIDS and,
        62-63
    churches' responses to, 62
    economic effects of, 64
    intravenous drug abuse-related
        transmission of, 51
    preventive interventions for,
        53-58,63-65
        community involvement
            theory-based, 53-54,64-65
        health beliefs model-based, 52-53
        reasoned action theory-based,
            52-53
        social cognitive learning
            theory-based, 52-53,64
    in prisons, 61
    sexual activity-related transmission of,
        51,52
        among Caribbean communities,
            55-58
        among Caribbean immigrants,
            58-62
        among tourism industry
            workers, 55-56
        interventions for prevention of,
            53-58
        relationship with social norms, 54
        socio-cultural factors in, 60-62
Holmes, Wendell, 158
Homosexuals, HIV/AIDS in,
    51,55,59-60,61-62
Human immunodeficiency virus (HIV)
    infection. *See* HIV/AIDS
Human rights, of immigrants, 151-152

Illegal Immigration Reform and
    Immigrant Responsibility Act
    of 1996, 84-85

Elite Preference Policy Analysis of,
    149-150,151,152,155-161,
    163,165
    implication for domestic violence
        prevention, 130-132
    implication for U. S. immigration
        policy, 161-163
Immigrants
    criminal behavior of, 151
    educational level of, 151
    female
        Afro-Caribbean, 13. *See also*
            Caribbean immigrant women;
            West Indian older immigrant
            women
        as percentage of total
            international migration, 13
    human rights of, 151-152
    poverty rate among, 151
    unemployed status of, 151
Immigrant's Journal, 70
Immigration and Nationality Act of
    1965, 150
Immigration policy
    government's responsibility for,
        151
    implication for domestic violence
        prevention, 1301-32
    implication for older West Indian
        immigrant women, 25
    post-September 11, 2001,
        76-77,79-80
    toward Caribbean countries, 163
Immigration Reform and Control Act
    of 1996. *See* Illegal
        Immigration Reform and
        Immigrant Responsibility Act
        of 1996
Immigration Reform of 1965, 2
Incarceration, of immigrants, 156
Infant mortality, 29-48
    among Caribbean immigrants in
        New York City, 32-45
    effects of cultural beliefs and
        practices on, 35,39-42

effects of English-language
deficiencies on, 37,40-41,44
effects of perinatal health care
on, 35,36,39,41-42,43,44
focus group studies of,
35-36,39-41,44-45
Health Keepers Model of
intervention for, 44
recommended interventions for,
44-45
among people of color, 31-32
as health status indicator, 30-31
international comparison of, 31
main causes of, 42-43
International Labor Organization, 152
Intravenous drug abusers, HIV/AIDS
in, 51,60

Jamaica
annual migration from, 2-3
criminal immigrants' repatriation
to, 158
deportation negotiations with the
United States, 78
female-headed households in, 137
HIV/AIDS in
among children, 58
misconceptions about, 62-63
immigrants' remittances to, 3
Jamaica AIDS Support, 55
Jamaican Daily Gleaner, 158
Jamaican immigrants
female-headed households of, 137
infant mortality rate among,
39,40-41
in New York City, 3
refusal of repatriation by, 160
Joint United Nations Program on
HIV/AIDS, 50-51

Labor rights, 152
Latinas, psychological effects of
migration in, 86

Latinos, opposition to immigration
legislation, 159
Levin, Sander, 155
Low birth weight, 31-32

March on Washington (1996), 159
Massachusetts, domestic violence
policy in, 118
Medicaid, 153,154,155
Medicare, 21,23
Migration, rationale for, 85-86
Migration-related decision-making
processes, in Caribbean
women, 83-101
during acculturation, 93-97
active planning process, 89
active preparation process, 91
conscious awareness process, 88-89
critical thinking process, 90-91
grief, 88-89,97,98
internal struggling, 95-97
during migration, 91-93
prior to migration, 87-91
relief and hope, 94-95
resolve, 97
subconscious awareness process,
87,88
support network development,
85,89-90,96,97
Miller, Jean Baker, 105
Minority groups, as percentage of total
U.S. population, 12
Mothering, transnational, 95-96
Moynihan, Daniel Patrick, 155

National Asian Pacific American Legal
Consortium, 159
National Center for Health Statistics,
31,42
National Center for Injury Prevention
and Control, 104
Nevis, annual migration from, 2
New York City

Caribbean immigrants in
    HIV/AIDS prevalence in, 58-60
    infant mortality rates among,
        32-45
    population of, 3-4
    foreign-born and immigrant
        populations in, 36,37,84
    gender analysis of, 84-85
    HIV/AIDS among
        African-American
        homosexuals in, 59-60
    Jamaican female-headed
        households in, 137
New York State
    domestic violence policy in, 118
    number of undocumented
        immigrants in, 84
New York Times, 72
Nigerian immigrants, infant mortality
    rate among, 40
Non-Citizen Benefit Clarification and
    Other Technical Amendment
    Act of 1998, 154
Northern California Coalition for
    Immigrants, 159
Norway, infant mortality rate in, 31

Oklahoma City, federal building
    bombing in (1995), 152

Pakistanian immigrants, infant
    mortality rate among, 40
Panamanian immigrants, infant
    mortality rate among, 39,40
Parent-child relationships, of
        Caribbean and West Indian
        immigrant families
    during adolescence, 106-107
    discipline issues in, 137-138
    effect of separation and
        reunification on, 138-139
    during acculturation, 93-97
    during migration, 91-93
    prior to migration, 88-91
    social services interventions for,
        141
Parenting style, of West Indians,
        137-138
"Partnership with America," 149
Patriot Act, 76
Personal Responsibility and Work
        Reconciliation Act of 1996,
        25
    Elite Preference Policy Analysis of,
        149-150,152,153-155
    impact on immigrant families,
        153-154
    institutional response to, 154-155
Peruvian immigrants, infant mortality
    rate among, 40
Political power, of immigrants, 164
Population, of the U.S.
    Caribbean immigrants as
        percentage of, 164
    foreign-born, 164
    older West Indians as percentage of,
        13
    racial and ethnic demographics of,
        12
Posttraumatic stress disorder, 73
Poverty
    of immigrants, 151
    of West Indian New York City
        communities, 5
Powell, Colin, 161
Powerlessness, 142-143
Pregnancy, HIV/AIDS transmission
        during, 57,58
Prisons, 152-153. *See also*
        Incarceration
    HIV/AIDS transmission within, 61
Prostitutes, HIV/AIDS in, 58
Psychiatric illness
    among Caribbean immigrants, 4
    among deported immigrants,
        158-159

Public services and benefits. *See* Social
   services and benefits
Puerto Rican immigrants, infant
   mortality rate among, 39,40

Racial profiling, 76-77,79
Racism, toward Caribbean immigrants,
   4,5,94
Restraining orders, 118,119
   in Barbados (Domestic Violence
      Act), 119-120,122,125
   effectiveness of, 125-130
   men's hostility toward,
      122,123-124

St. Cyr, Enrico, 162
St. Kitts, annual migration from, 2
St. Vincent, HIV/AIDS-related deaths
   in, 55
School-based prevention model, for
   dating violence, 107-115
   intervention group component of,
      111-112
   parent/community awareness
      component of, 111
   school staff awareness component
      of, 110-111
   student awareness component of,
      109-110
   young men's early intervention
      group component of, 112-114
   young women's early intervention
      group component of, 114-115
School-related problems, of West
   Indian immigrant children,
   5,136,140
Segregation, residential, 4-5
Separation
   of immigrant families, implication
      for sexual relations, 60-61
   parent-child. *See also* Child
      fostering

Separation and individuation, role in
   gender identity development,
   105
September 11, 2001. *See also* World
   Trade Center tragedy
   Caribbean women immigrants'
      emotional reactions to, 93
September 11 Fund, 80
Sex tourism, 55-56
Sexual behavior, as HIV/AIDS risk
   factor, 51,52
   among Caribbean communities,
      55-58
   among Caribbean immigrants,
      58-62
   among child prostitutes, 58
   among tourism industry workers,
      55-56
   gender factors in, 63
   misconceptions about, 62-63
   preventive intervention models for,
      53-58,63-65
      community intervention model,
         53-54,64-65
      reasoned action theory-based,
         52-53
      social cognitive theory-based,
         52-53,64
   relationship with social norms, 54
Sexually transmitted diseases, in
   Caribbean immigrants, 59
Skilled workers, U.S. immigration
   policy toward, 163
Socialization, into gender roles, 105
Social Security Disability (SSDI),
   21-22,23
Social services and benefits. *See also*
   Food stamps; Medicaid;
   Medicare; Social Security
   Disability (SSDI);
   Supplemental Social Security
   (SSI)
   Caribbean immigrants' utilization
      of

among older West Indian
women immigrants, 20-26
legislative restrictions on, 153
post-September 11, 2001, 79
Social support networks, of Caribbean
immigrant women,
85,89-90,96,97
Social work, with West Indian
immigrants, 135-145
family conflict/stress issues in,
136-140
child rearing practices, 137-138
employment, 139-140,141
family relationships, 137
parent-adolescent relationship,
106-107
parent-child separation and
reunification (child
fostering), 138-139
school-related problems,
5,136,140
multilevel approach in, 140-143
advocacy in, 141,142
empowerment in, 141,142-143
referrals in, 136
Stewart, Kendall, 72
Stigmatization, of people with
HIV/AIDS, 63-64
Sudden infant death syndrome (SIDS),
32,42
Supplemental Social Security (SSI),
21-22,23,153
Sweden, infant mortality rate in, 31
Syphilis, 59

Temporary Assistance to Needy
Families, 153
Tourism industry workers, HIV/AIDS
prevalence among, 55
Trinidad and Tobago
HIV/AIDS prevalence in, 57
immigrants from
infant mortality rate among, 40
in New York City, 3

Trinidad and Tobago Rape Centre, 124

Unemployment insurance program, of
the September 11, Fund, 80
United Nations Children Fund
(UNICEF), 58
United States Department of
Homeland Security,
71,76,160
United States Immigration and
Naturalization Services
(INS), as part of Department
of Homeland Security, 160
University of the West Indies, 158
Urban Institute, 25

Velazquez, Nydia, 159
Violence Against Women Act
(VAWA), 131
Visiting Nurses Services, New York
City, 74

Welfare policy, implications for older
West Indian immigrant
women, 25
Welfare Reform Act. *See* Personal
Responsibility and Work
Reconciliation Act of 1996
West Indian immigrants
"Black Success" model of, 18,25
documented, 2
failure to utilize welfare benefits,
154
family structure of, 137,138
in New York City, 3
social services underutilization by,
136
sources of family conflict/stress in,
136-140
child rearing practices, 137-138
employment, 139-140,141

family relationships, 137
parent-child separation and
reunification, 138-139
school-related problems,
5,136,140
West Indian men
gender-based roles of, 137
social status of, 140
West Indian older women immigrants,
11-28
residing in Greater Hartford,
Connecticut, 14-25
demographic characteristics of,
16-18
disabling conditions among,
20,21-22,23,24
effect of aging policy on, 25,26
effect of immigration and
welfare policies on, 25
health status of, 19-20,21
incomes of, 17,18-19,25
income sources of, 21-22
poverty of,
17,18-19,21-22,23,24
socioeconomic characteristics
of, 16-18
underutilization of community
benefits and services by,
20-26

West Indian people, definition of, 2
West Indian women, gender-based
roles of, 137
World Bank Report, 57
World Trade Center tragedy, effects on
Caribbean immigrants, 69-82
detention and deportation, 72,75,78
discrimination and harassment,
71-72
immigration policy changes,
76-77,79-80
loss of life, 70-71,79
psychological stress reactions,
72-73,75-76,77-79
coping strategies for, 77,78-79
racial profiling, 76-77,79
social workers' responses to,
70,72,74,77-78,79-81

Zadvydas v. *Davis,* 160

BOOK ORDER FORM!

Order a copy of this book with this form or online at:
http://www.haworthpress.com/store/product.asp?sku=5352

The Health and Well-Being of Caribbean Immigrants in the United States

_____ in softbound at $24.95 (ISBN: 0-7890-0446-1)
_____ in hardbound at $49.95 (ISBN: 0-7890-0442-9)

COST OF BOOKS _____

POSTAGE & HANDLING _____
US: $4.00 for first book & $1.50
for each additional book.
Outside US: $5.00 for first book
& $2.00 for each additional book.

SUBTOTAL _____

In Canada: add 7% GST. _____

STATE TAX _____
CA, IL, IN, MN, NJ, NY, OH & SD residents
please add appropriate local sales tax.

FINAL TOTAL _____
If paying in Canadian funds, convert
using the current exchange rate,
UNESCO coupons welcome.

❑BILL ME LATER:
Bill-me option is good on US/Canada/
Mexico orders only; not good to jobbers,
wholesalers, or subscription agencies.

❑ Signature _____

❑ Payment Enclosed: $ _____

❑ PLEASE CHARGE TO MY CREDIT CARD:
❑ Visa ❑ MasterCard ❑ AmEx ❑ Discover
❑ Diner's Club ❑ Eurocard ❑ JCB

Account # _____

Exp Date _____

Signature _____
(Prices in US dollars and subject to change without notice.)

PLEASE PRINT ALL INFORMATION OR ATTACH YOUR BUSINESS CARD
Name
Address
City   State/Province   Zip/Postal Code
Country
Tel   Fax
E-Mail

May we use your e-mail address for confirmations and other types of information? ❑Yes ❑No We appreciate receiving
your e-mail address. Haworth would like to e-mail special discount offers to you, as a preferred customer.
We will never share, rent, or exchange your e-mail address. We regard such actions as an invasion of your privacy.

Order From Your **Local Bookstore** or Directly From
The Haworth Press, Inc. 10 Alice Street, Binghamton, New York 13904-1580 • USA
Call Our toll-free number (1-800-429-6784) / Outside US/Canada: (607) 722-5857
Fax: 1-800-895-0582 / Outside US/Canada: (607) 771-0012
E-mail your order to us: orders@haworthpress.com

For orders outside US and Canada, you may wish to order through your local
sales representative, distributor, or bookseller.
For information, see http://haworthpress.com/distributors

(Discounts are available for individual orders in US and Canada only, not booksellers/distributors.)

Please photocopy this form for your personal use.
www.HaworthPress.com

BOF04